Positioning the
Surgical Patient

To our wives, with thanks for their
patience, forbearance and understanding

Positioning the Surgical Patient

J. M. ANDERTON, FFARCS
Consultant Anaesthetist, Manchester Royal Infirmary

R. I. KEEN, FFARCS
Consultant Anaesthetist, Manchester Royal Infirmary

R. NEAVE, FMAA
Medical Artist, University of Manchester

Butterworths
London   Boston   Singapore   Sydney   Toronto   Wellington

First published, 1988

© **J. M. Anderton, R. I. Keen and R. Neave, 1988**

British Library Cataloguing in Publication Data

Anderton, J. M.
  Positioning the surgical patient.
  1. Position (Surgery)
  I. Title II. Keen, R. I. III. Neave, R.
  617′.91   RD32.7

ISBN 0-407-01220-6

Library of Congress Cataloging-in-Publication Data

Anderton, J. M.
  Positioning the surgical patient.
  Includes index.
  1. Position (Surgery) I. Keen, R. I. II. Neave, R.
III. Title.
RD32.7.A53 1988   617′.91′028   87-22433

ISBN 0-407-01220-6

Photoset by Butterworths Litho Preparation Department
Printed and bound in Great Britain by
Anchor Brendon Ltd., Tiptree, Essex

Foreword

Before the Second World War textbooks on anaesthetics invariably included a section dealing with the positioning of the patient on the operating table for various types of surgery. They not only described how each position was achieved, but warned against the hazards which were associated with it. However, surgery has become ever more complex and extensive, and the positions (or contortions), into which the patient's body now has to be manoeuvred to accommodate the surgical operation concerned, also get more complicated; but this important aspect of anaesthesia has gradually received less attention in the textbooks. Yet, these positions have the propensity for great harm, and they have indeed led to serious physical and physiological injuries. That cardinal guide to all medical practice, and especially to anaesthesia, 'Primum non nocere' (Above all do no harm!), is in danger of being forgotten. It is therefore refreshing to see that Drs Anderton and Keen, two of my former pupils and associates, have seriously and diligently collected into what will surely become a standard reference and instructional book, all that is known about the positioning of patients for surgery. They describe in great detail how each position is achieved, the problems it poses for safe anaesthesia, and the precautions which must be taken to avoid injury. It is virtually impossible to organize prospective experimental studies of these hazards, for that would involve serious ethical problems. There is fortunately a considerable literature, mostly of an anecdotal nature, in which it should be noted, the authors' own experience forms a not inconsiderable part. *In toto*, there is now a very clear picture of the incidence and prevention of these injuries.

The two clinical authors were fortunate in getting the collaboration of Mr R. Neave as co-author. He is an unusually expert and sensitive artist, and his beautiful and accurate drawings make doubly clear what even the best text sometimes leaves in doubt.

This book is not just for anaesthetists. The duty of care for the whole patient is shared between anaesthetist and surgeon, each with his own well defined skills and areas of responsibility. Surgeons will therefore also read this book with interest and advantage. So too will those, both in and outside the medical profession who, regrettably, have to deal with the almost inevitable medicolegal consequences when these injuries occur. Others who work in operating rooms and intensive care units, such as nurses and technicians, should also have access to this book, for they too, within their spheres of competence may be asked or even be expected to share some of the responsibility with doctors, for the care of patients. In short this book will have a wide appeal, and I sincerely hope it will become mandatory reading for all who have the welfare of the surgical patient at heart.

William W. Mushin, CBE, MA, DSc, FRCS, FFARCS
Emeritus Professor of Anaesthetics
University of Wales College of Medicine

Preface

The original concept of this book was to provide a clear-cut set of well illustrated instructions on the positioning of patients for various forms of surgery. The second objective was to describe the hazards involved, in an attempt to improve safety for the patient. It soon became obvious that readers might wish to consult original sources, and we have therefore produced a reasonably full set of references.

Each chapter has been set out in a similar format; hazards, anaesthetic considerations and technique. The physiological changes involved in positioning patients are complex and, in order to avoid repetition, have been dealt with in a separate chapter. Although it should be of interest to anaesthetists, it may be regarded as an 'optional extra' for other members of the theatre team.

The illustrations are mainly drawn to highlight one or two particular points; for simplicity, other aspects mentioned in the text may well have been omitted although they appear in adjacent illustrations.

The techniques of positioning described, largely reflect the authors' (JMA/RIK) own experience and practice. The sitting position is, however, one with which we are not recently familiar. We have been fortunate in persuading Dr T. V. Campkin to write this chapter. Greater details of anaesthetic technique and monitoring have been included than are to be found in other chapters, but because of the potential dangers of this position, we feel that this is entirely appropriate. We also acknowledge the late Dr J. V. I. Young's help with the description of the air evacuation mattress given in Chapter 7 and express our sadness that he was not able to review the published work.

We are grateful to all our colleagues who have so readily offered advice and assistance in the preparation of this book. Professor T. E. J. Healy has both encouraged us and loaned us a valuable selection of reprints. A number of consultant colleagues have read and commented critically on the script at various stages of preparation. Surgeons and theatre staff have helped us with their patience, forbearance and advice. The photographers who provided much of the reference work for the illustrations have provided an incomparable and efficient service.

The departmental secretaries, in particular Mrs Kathy Dimelow, have dealt with the task cheerfully and promptly, despite seemingly ever changing texts.

Finally we want to thank Mr Charles Fry of Butterworths for patient guidance and Professor W. W. Mushin, mentor in our formative years, for agreeing to write the Foreword.

J. M. Anderton
R. I. Keen
R. Neave

Contents

Chapter one

The supine position

Almost all patients presenting for surgery have anaesthesia induced in the supine position; a very high proportion also remain in this position for their operation. This is fortunate because minimal manipulation of the patient is required, the physiological upset is small and the anatomical hazards are easily avoided.

Unfortunately, however, it must be stressed that any unconscious, supine patient is at risk of aspirating gastric contents into the lungs. This is a serious life-threatening hazard and remains a major cause of morbidity and mortality (Utting, Gray and Shelley, 1979; DHSS, 1982). Anaesthesia must never be induced in the supine patient unless the operating table or trolley is capable of being tipped rapidly into the head-down position. Efficient suction apparatus must also be at hand. At the completion of surgery the patient should always be turned into the lateral position unless there is a specific contraindication to this.

Anatomical hazards

These usually result from abnormal external pressure, traction or inappropriate joint movements. Interference with the very delicate blood vessels supplying the nerves is probably the principal factor in the majority of peripheral nerve injuries. Only 30 to 40 minutes of anaesthesia in an unfavourable posture may be sufficient to produce a nerve palsy (Britt and Gordon, 1964). From above downwards the hazards are as follows:

(1) The supra-orbital nerve can be compressed by nasal endotracheal tube connectors if insufficient padding is used (Barrow, 1955) (*Figure 1.1*).

(2) External pressure on the eyes can easily occur from a badly fitting face-mask. Initially, this will cause a reduction in intra-ocular pressure but will be followed, postoperatively,

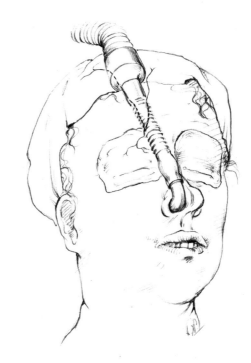

Figure 1.1 Pressure on the supra-orbital nerve from endotracheal tube connector

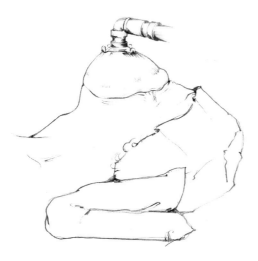
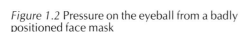

Figure 1.2 Pressure on the eyeball from a badly positioned face mask

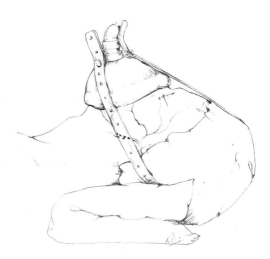

Figure 1.3 Pressure on branch of the facial nerve from a tight face-mask harness

by a rise in tension above the normal. The latter may persist for several hours and it has been suggested that glaucoma may be precipitated in a susceptible patient (Brittain and Brittain, 1945) (*Figure 1.2*).

In patients with an intra-ocular lens implant there are particular mechanical risks from any form of external pressure on the eyeball. Displacement of the implant with or without secondary damage to the cornea, or intra-ocular haemorrhage, may result.

The cornea should never be left exposed. There are the obvious risks of mechanical trauma, contamination with corrosive fluids such as skin antiseptics, aerosol sprayed wound dressings and regurgitated gastric acid. Less obvious is the risk of corneal drying; 10 minutes' exposure without eyelid movement is sufficient to produce surface dehydration. Epithelial breakdown, infection and permanent corneal scarring can then occur. Patients from special care units, often harbouring virulent organisms and having diminished powers of protection seem to be at greatest risk.

(3) Branches of the facial nerve may be compressed by a tightly applied face-mask harness or a tape used to secure the endo-tracheal tube (Fuller and Thomas, 1956) (*Figure 1.3*).

(4) Traction injury to the brachial plexus is a well recognized complication related to body position (Lincoln and Sawyer, 1961). Its anatomical fixation in the neck and axilla and its close proximity to the bony structures of the clavicle, first rib and head of the humerus are predisposing factors (*Figure 1.4*). Abduction to 90 degrees should only be permitted providing the hand is pronated and the head is turned towards the abducted arm (*Figure 1.5*). This minimizes tension on the nerve roots. Arm retainers must always be in position before anaesthesia is induced to prevent the arms from falling down at loss of consciousness. This precaution prevents traction injury to the brachial plexus as well as damage to the shoulder joint capsular ligaments.

(5) The radial nerve spiralling round the humerus is poorly protected and can easily be damaged by external pressure from a screen (*Figure 1.6a*).

(6) The ulnar nerve in its groove behind the medial epicondyle can be damaged if allowed to be compressed by the edge of the mattress (*Figure 1.6b*).

(7) Failure to provide support for the normal lumbosacral curvature may be a cause of postoperative backache (*Figure 1.7*). The use of

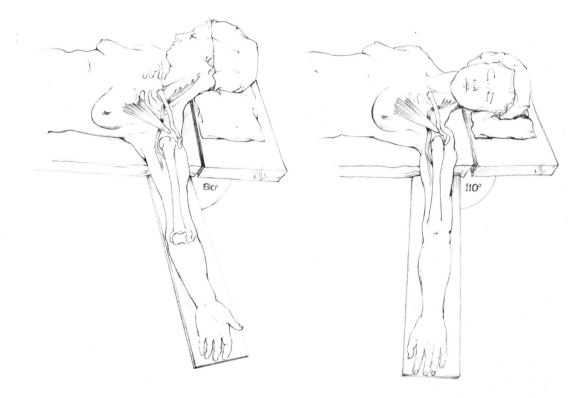

Figure 1.4 Traction on the brachial plexus from incorrect position of arm and head

Figure 1.5 Correct position of arm and head

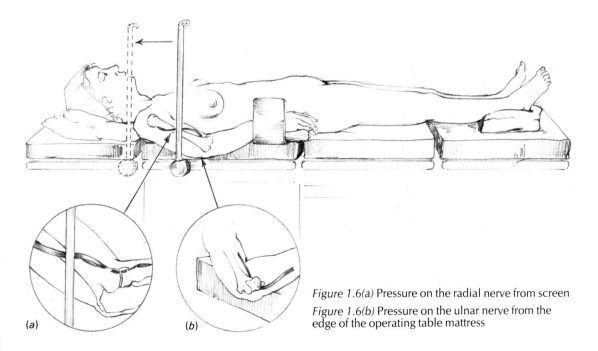

Figure 1.6(a) Pressure on the radial nerve from screen

Figure 1.6(b) Pressure on the ulnar nerve from the edge of the operating table mattress

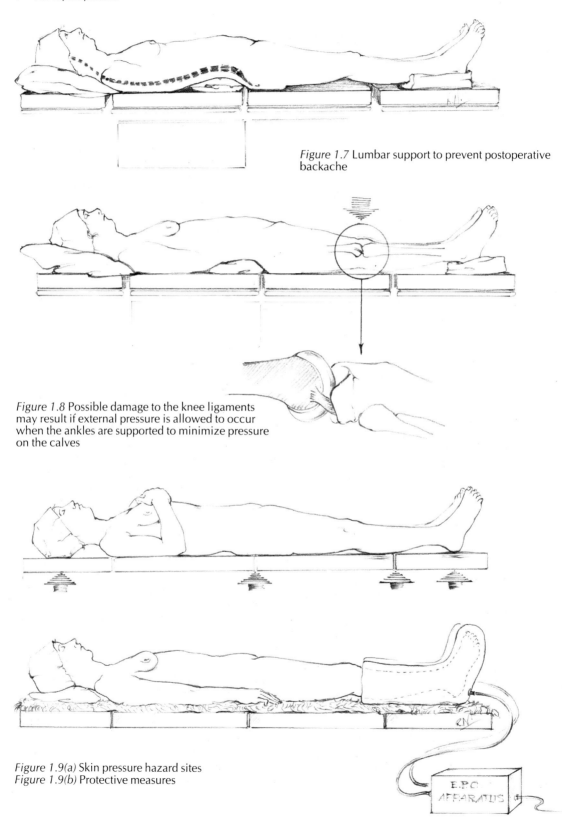

Figure 1.7 Lumbar support to prevent postoperative backache

Figure 1.8 Possible damage to the knee ligaments may result if external pressure is allowed to occur when the ankles are supported to minimize pressure on the calves

Figure 1.9(a) Skin pressure hazard sites
Figure 1.9(b) Protective measures

E.P.C APPARATUS

an inflatable wedge has been shown to reduce significantly the incidence of this complication (O'Donovan *et al.,* 1986).

(8) Hyperextension injury to the knee or damage to the internal cruciate ligaments is a theoretical risk if the ankles have been supported on foam pads (*see below*) (*Figure 1.8*). This is certainly not a comfortable position for the conscious patient to maintain and as such should probably be avoided. The risk is enhanced if surgical or nursing assistants inadvertently lean across the legs. Although there do not appear to be any reports of such knee injuries in the medical literature, common sense dictates that care should be taken in this respect.

(9) Pressure necrosis to the skin over the occiput, sacrum and heel may occur unless they are properly padded (*Figure 1.9*). Usually the head is supported by a soft pillow and problems are fortunately rare. Postoperative pressure alopecia has been reported however following prolonged operations in which the blood pressure was deliberately lowered (Abel and Lewis, 1960). The various special head-rests, e.g. the horseshoe, are particularly hazardous, especially if surgical pressure is applied as frequently happens in aural or neurosurgical operations. The sacral skin is most easily protected by having a sheepskin rug between the patient and the mattress of the operating table. Pressure on the calf muscles of the lower legs may predispose to deep vein thrombosis and its inherent risk of pulmonary embolism. Similarly, the skin of the posterior aspect of the ankles may be damaged by pressure. In the past it has been common to support the Achilles tendons with a foam rubber pad in an attempt to solve both these problems. More recently, the use of external pneumatic compression (EPC) apparatus has been shown to be a significant advance in this field (Hirsch, 1981; Borow and Goldson, 1981) and is worthy of more widespread application. In the authors' experience, it is very easy for the lower limbs to be neglected, especially in operating theatres where short procedures are usual. If the patient lies throughout the operation with legs crossed both calves are compressed, as are the underlying long saphenous vein and dorsalis pedis artery; clearly this should never be allowed to happen (*Figure 1.10*).

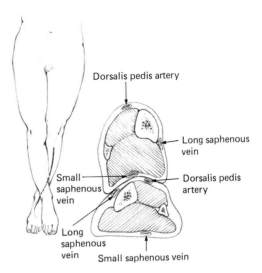

Figure 1.10 Important structures compressed by crossed legs

Preliminary preparation

Placing the patient in position for a surgical operation usually requires 'team-effort'. The anaesthetist generally directs operations by virtue of holding the responsibility for the patient's safety and wellbeing. Operating room assistants, who are often very skilled and experienced, carry out the necessary man-oeuvres and the surgeon approves or modifies the final position. When more complicated operations are scheduled or special instruments, such as the operating microscope, are to be used it is customary for the surgeon to supervise the final stages personally. It is essential that there should be adequate access around the patient for all the necessary man-oeuvres to be performed safely. The assistants must be present in sufficient numbers and have the requisite strength to deal with the size of patient presented. Above all, they should understand the steps of the positioning man-oeuvre to be performed. Finally it is important that all the ancillary equipment such as arm-rests, foam support pads, extra pillows, etc, have all been assembled together prior to starting the procedure.

Positioning for the induction of anaesthesia

The important prerequisites for the induction of anaesthesia in the supine position have already been mentioned at the beginning of this chapter. Except in some small children and very ill patients, anaesthesia is usually induced intravenously. Upper limb veins are almost invariably used and the arm concerned may be supported separately on an arm-board or retained close to the patient's side. Both arms must be adequately secured prior to loss of consciousness to prevent them falling off the table.

Following intravenous induction, anaesthesia may be maintained with volatile agents via a face-mask. It is important that this is positioned correctly so that a good seal is obtained against the skin of the face. There are two basic patterns of face-mask in common use. Their main difference is in the positioning of their lower rim in relation to the mandible (*Figure 1.11*). If the face-mask is to be retained in position with a harness, it must be remembered that too tight an application may damage branches of the facial nerve and that the orbital structures must be avoided.

Correct positioning of the head for endotracheal intubation

The patient's head and neck must be supported on a pillow which must not extend beneath the shoulders. There should thus be good forward flexion of the neck and extension of the head at the atlanto-occipital joint. This position has been described as 'sniffing the morning air' (*Figure 1.12*). This was almost certainly first described by Alfred Kirstein (Kirstein, 1886;

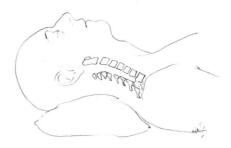

Figure 1.12 Correctly positioned pillow ensures flexion of the neck with extension of the head at the atlanto-occipital joint

Figure 1.11 Correct positioning of the lower rim of the face-mask depends on the pattern used

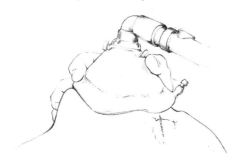

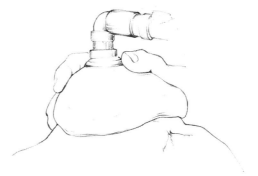

Hirsch, Smith and Hirsch, 1986) although for many years credit for it has been given to Chevalier Jackson (Jackson, 1907) a noted early otolaryngologist. It is important to pay attention to detail and place all patients for intubation in this position. Correct positioning will make some of the very difficult intubations possible. The risk of unexpected impossible intubation in a prospective series of Caesarean section patients has recently been reported as 1:300 (Lyons, 1985). It is possible to demonstrate the effectiveness of correct positioning for intubation by commencing laryngoscopy with the patient's head flat on the table. An assistant then gently raises the head-end of the table through approximately 30 degrees and the larynx will be seen to come into view (*Figure 1.13*). It may be argued that many anaesthetists apparently manage to intubate quite easily without carefully positioning the patient's head. This is simply because they are skilled and the intubations are not difficult. It is not an argument against the correct preparation.

The 'adult' position described above requires modification when neonates and small children are to be intubated. This is because the size of the head relative to the body aligns the cervical vertebrae naturally in the flexed position. Indeed, occasionally it may be necessary to put a small pad or pillow under the shoulders in order to get the axis right (*Figure 1.14*).

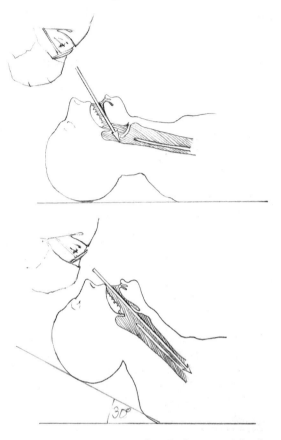

Figure 1.13 Failure to visualize the larynx with badly positioned head can be corrected by elevation

Figure 1.14 Intubation in neonates or small infants may sometimes be facilitated by a pillow under the shoulders

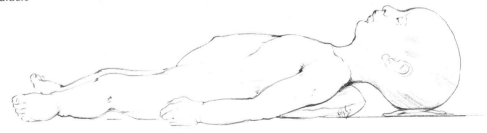

Correct positioning for the application of cricoid pressure

This manoeuvre was originally described by Sellick (1961) and is used in any situation when induction of anaesthesia carries a greater than normal risk of regurgitation of gastric contents. It is now an accepted part of the 'rapid-sequence induction' technique and it is always preceded by a period of pre-oxygenation for the patient. The principle makes use of the fact that the cricoid cartilage is the only tracheal ring which is complete around its entire circumference (*Figure 1.15*). Pressure on the anterior aspect will therefore compress the underlying oesophagus. It has recently been stressed (DHSS, 1986) that counter-pressure provided by a hand or forearm behind the neck should also be applied This is necessary to prevent the

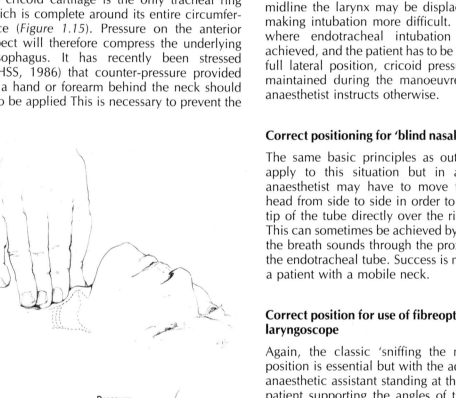

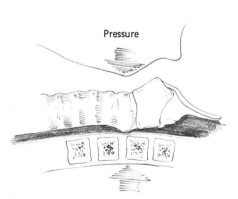

Pressure

Counter pressure

Figure 1.15 Cricoid pressure

head from becoming flexed and thereby making the intubation more difficult. It is essential that the assistant fully understands the exact site of the cricoid cartilage, starts compression when instructed by the anaesthetist and does not release pressure until the cuff of the endotracheal tube has been satisfactorily inflated. It cannot be stressed too strongly that misplaced 'cricoid' pressure applied over the laryngeal cartilages cannot properly seal the oesophagus; furthermore, if not applied directly in the midline the larynx may be displaced laterally making intubation more difficult. In situations where endotracheal intubation cannot be achieved, and the patient has to be turned to the full lateral position, cricoid pressure must be maintained during the manoeuvre unless the anaesthetist instructs otherwise.

Correct positioning for 'blind nasal' intubation

The same basic principles as outlined above apply to this situation but in addition the anaesthetist may have to move the patient's head from side to side in order to position the tip of the tube directly over the rima glottidis. This can sometimes be achieved by listening for the breath sounds through the proximal end of the endotracheal tube. Success is most likely in a patient with a mobile neck.

Correct position for use of fibreoptic laryngoscope

Again, the classic 'sniffing the morning air' position is essential but with the addition of an anaesthetic assistant standing at the side of the patient supporting the angles of the jaw. The purpose of this is to ensure that the tip of the laryngoscope passes from the mouth or nose into an open pharyngeal area. It should then be possible to visualize the larynx at the bottom of this space. Failure to hold the jaw forward results in the mucous membranes of the pharyngeal wall becoming approximated and all that can be seen through the laryngoscope is a pink blur.

Correct position for bronchoscopy

Occasionally, the anaesthetist has to resort to bronchoscopy using a rigid bronchoscope. First

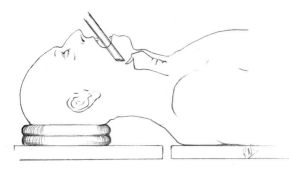

Figure 1.16 Initial position for insertion of rigid bronchoscope

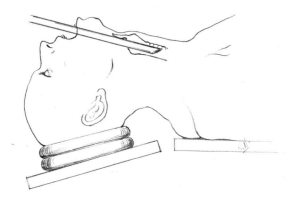

Figure 1.17 Further passage of the instrument cannot be achieved without extension of the neck

it is necessary to ensure that the patient is positioned with the level of the shoulders at the top 'break-point' of the operating table. A small pillow is placed under the neck and occiput. After introducing the bronchoscope in the midline and visualizing the epiglottis (*Figure 1.16*), the head section of the operating table is sufficiently lowered to enable the proximal end of the bronchoscope to assume a horizontal position and be advanced into the trachea (*Figure 1.17*).

Positioning and security of the endotracheal tube and its connections

There are many hazards related to the use of endotracheal tubes and a comprehensive discussion would be inappropriate. However, some of the more serious misadventures are related to the process of positioning the patient and discussion of these is pertinent. With increasing use of muscle relaxant drugs and strong respiratory depressant analgesics, failure to maintain the integrity of the airway or the connections to a means of artificial ventilation can produce irreversible brain-damaging hypoxia within a space of 3 to 5 minutes. There are four main possibilities related to position and security of the endotracheal tube.

(1) A tube initially correctly placed in the trachea may be further advanced into the right main bronchus (*Figure 1.18*). This will result in shunting 50 per cent of the pulmonary blood flow from right to the left side of the heart without the relevant gas exchange. Total atelectasis of the unaerated lung will eventually ensue. This complication of intubation is most likely to occur when head and neck surgery is being performed and may be a consequence of head movement at the time the surgical drapes are applied. It may also result from pressure applied directly to the catheter mount or endotracheal tube by nursing or surgical assistants who rarely have any appreciation or regard for anaesthetic apparatus beneath the drapes.

(2) The endotracheal tube can be pulled out of the larynx and come out altogether. This is usually due both to improper securement at the face and to excessive traction by the breathing hoses.

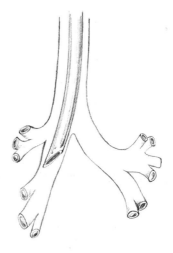

Figure 1.18 Almost straight alignment of the right main bronchus favours entry of an endotracheal tube advanced beyond the carina

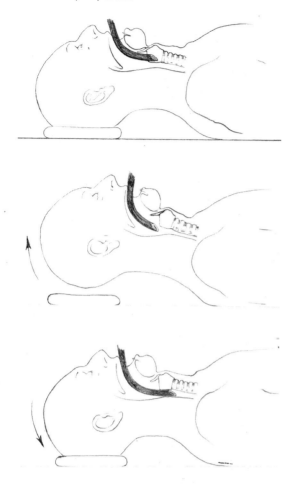

Figure 1.19 Inadvertent extubation of a short endotracheal tube can follow head manipulation. It may then lie in the pharynx or enter the oesophagus

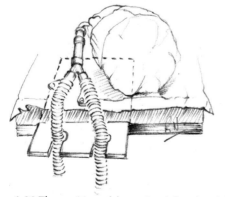

Figure 1.20 The position of the patient's head and the breathing hose supports must minimize tension and possible disruption of airway continuity

(3) The endotracheal tube, especially if rather short, can be pulled out of the larynx when head towels are being applied, but then slip into the oesophagus when the head is repositioned. This hazard is more difficult to diagnose quickly and accurately (*Figure 1.19*).

(4) The endotracheal tube can remain correctly sited but a disconnection on either the inspiratory or expiratory limb of the breathing circuit can occur. The resultant massive gas leak from the circuit will result in total failure of lung ventilation.

There is an obvious case for the use of ventilator or disconnection alarms in all patients on intermittent positive pressure ventilation (IPPV), but attention to detail in the securing of the endotracheal tubes is of equal importance. Irrespective of the method used, the stability and position of the patient's head in relation to the breathing hose connections is critical (*Figure 1.20*). All such connections should be held firmly in position, and the possibility of unexpected traction should be anticipated.

Final adjustments to supine position for surgery

Following the successful induction of anaesthesia it is important that any further infusions or monitoring catheters should be inserted whilst the patient is still in the anaesthetic room. Surgeons impatient to start the operation are thereby kept at a distance so that they do not distract the anaesthetist. Martin (1978) has drawn attention to the fact that poor supine positioning can initiate a cycle of patient discomfort and agitation which may terminate surgery performed under regional blockade. It is essential, therefore, to treat patients under general anaesthesia with greater consideration than simply to leave them supine on a flat operating table. For comfort, the use of lumbar support wedges and EPC apparatus for the legs may be of some help. A more widespread use of the 'lawn chair position' (Martin, 1978) should be considered (*Figure 1.21*). This distributes support along the full length of the dorsal body surface and also permits gentle flexion of the hips and knees, placing them in more anatomically neutral positions.

Transfer to the operating room should be effected smoothly and quickly by staff fully conversant with the procedure. The anaesthetic

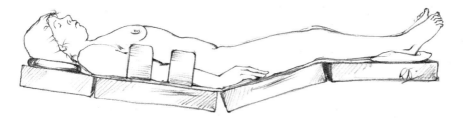

Figure 1.21 The lawn-chair position. (After Martin, 1978, with permission of the publishers)

Figure 1.22 Final operating position: supine with left arm on a board

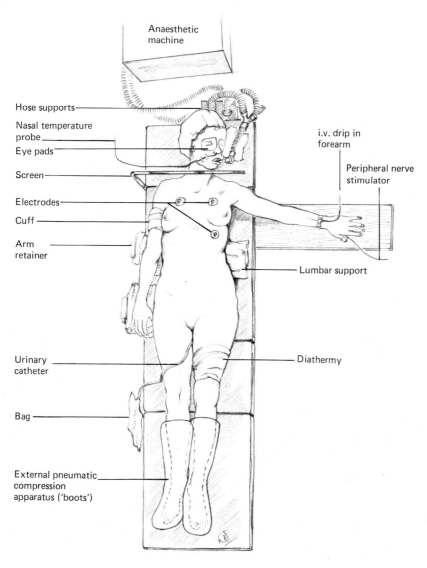

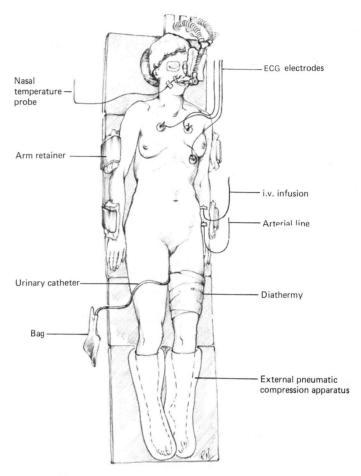

Nasal
temperature —
probe

ECG electrodes

Arm retainer —

i.v. infusion

Arterial line

Urinary catheter—

Diathermy

Bag —

External pneumatic
compression apparatus

Figure 1.23 Final operating position: supine with
arms at the side

machine and monitoring devices must be
reconnected with little delay. Whenever possible the anaesthetist should not permit the
patient's face to be covered by surgical towels.
A simple metal screen attached at the side of the
operating table can be placed transversely over
the patient at shoulder level. The drapes are
folded down across its cephalic aspect and thus
allow a good view of the patient's head. This
permits instant visual assurance of the continuity of airway connections and the identification
of subtle early changes in physiological parameters.

The final 'in theatre' supine position for
surgery will be covered by one of the following
three options:

(1) Supine with left arm on board (*Figure
1.22*);
(2) Supine with both arms at the sides (*Figure
1.23*);
(3) Supine with both arms folded across the
chest.

Some common modifications of the supine position

Slight head-down tilt

Here the patient remains supine and the table is
tilted approximately 20 degrees into the head-
down position. The legs remain fully extended.

It is used almost exclusively for lower limb surgery where tourniquets are not required and the rationale is reduction of bleeding at the operation site. Anatomically, all peripheral veins below heart level possess non-return valves and if the limb is raised above heart level, preferential flow will take the blood directly to the great veins. Its most common application is in the surgical correction of varicose veins.

The Trendelenburg position (Meyer, 1885; Trendelenburg, 1890) (*Figure 1.24*)

This consists of a much steeper degree of head-down tilt; approximately 35 to 40 degrees with the lowermost section of the operating table sometimes angled into the horizontal position. The knees are carefully positioned over this lower break in the table so that the legs provide some counter-traction against the tendency to slip cephalad. The construction of modern operating table mattresses with secure attachments to the table-top and non-slip upper surfaces has been of great value in this respect and may render knee flexion unnecessary. However, the risk remains, and can be accentuated if smooth stretcher covers or plastic water blankets are placed between the patient and mattress. Fortunately, nowadays, most enlight-

ened surgeons, mindful of the obvious physiological insult to the patient that this position imposes, do not request such steep degrees of tilt as were used formerly. The legs need not always be flexed and the shoulder retainers often seen in older texts on this subject are absolutely contraindicated. They present a positive danger to the brachial plexus (Ewing, 1950).

The Trendelenburg position is used almost exclusively for the abdominal approach to gynaecological and other pelvic surgery and uses gravity to assist in ensuring that the bowel is prevented from entering the surgical field. In the view of some authors (Inglis and Brook, 1956; Swain, 1960) the use of muscle relaxants in anaesthesia for abdominal surgery has rendered this position obsolete.

Anaesthetists should note that an adverse change in the position of the endotracheal tube can take place when the patient is tipped into the Trendelenburg position. Heinonen, Takki and Tammisto (1969) have shown that 40 per cent of patients have radiological evidence of upward displacement of the carina. In half of these, this will be sufficient to cause an endotracheal tube (previously positioned with the tip just above the carina) to enter the right main bronchus. It is, therefore, wise to check for adequate aeration of *both* sides of the chest after the patient has been positioned.

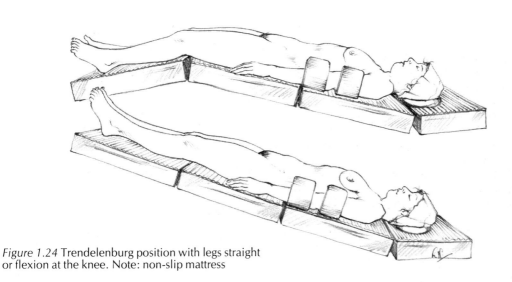

Figure 1.24 Trendelenburg position with legs straight or flexion at the knee. Note: non-slip mattress

Head-up tilt (reverse Trendelenburg)

This position is self-explanatory and varying degrees of tilt are employed. It is almost always used for major surgery on the head and neck region. Often in the latter quite steep degrees of tilt are used, but it is an easy matter to prevent the patient slipping caudally simply by the correct placement of a foot-rest at 90 degrees to the table-top (*Figure 1.25*).

The rationale for its use is to promote venous drainage away from the operating site and to assist in providing good operating conditions, particularly for intracranial, middle ear and plastic surgical procedures. It potentiates anaesthetic hypotensive techniques. The physiological implications are particularly relevant to the cardiovascular system and will be discussed later. Air embolism is also a serious risk.

Figure 1.25 Head-up position incorporating foot-rest

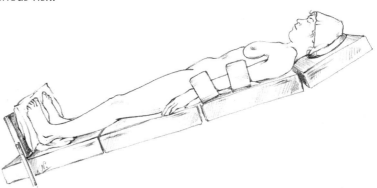

The supine position for hip replacement surgery

In order to provide good access to the operation site the patient is placed as near as possible to the lateral edge of the table.

The supine position for knee surgery

The patient remains supine but the lower section of the table is removed or rotated through 90 degrees and both knees are allowed to assume the flexed position. A pad is placed under the thigh on the operation side (*Figure 1.26*).

Figure 1.26 Position for meniscectomy

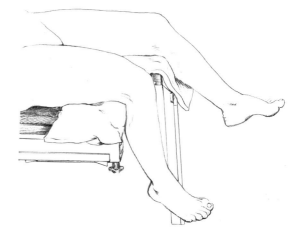

References

Abel, R. R. and Lewis, G. M. (1960) Postoperative (pressure) alopecia. *Archives of Dermatology*, **81**, 34–42

Barrow, D. W. (1955) Supraorbital neuropraxia. *Anaesthesia*, **10**, 374

Borow, M. and Goldson, H. (1981) Postoperative venous thrombosis. Evaluation of five methods of treatment. *American Journal of Surgery*, **141**, 245–251

Britt, B. A. and Gordon, R. A. (1964) Peripheral nerve injuries associated with anaesthesia. *Canadian Anaesthetists Society Journal*, **II**, 514–536

Brittain, I. and Brittain, G. J. C. (1945) Unilateral hypotony during anaesthesia. *British Medical Journal*, **1**, 442–444

Department of Health and Social Security (1982) Report on Confidential Enquiries into Maternal Deaths in England and Wales, 1976–1978. HMSO, London, **26**, 79–80

Department of Health and Social Security (1986) Report on Confidential Enquiries into Maternal Deaths in England and Wales, 1979–81. HMSO, London, **29**, 92

Ewing, M. R. (1950) Postoperative paralysis in the upper extremity. *Lancet*, **i**, 99–104

Fuller, J. E. and Thomas, D. V. (1956) Facial nerve paralysis after general anaesthesia. *Journal of American Medical Association*, **162**, 645

Heinonen, J., Takki, S. and Tammisto, T. (1969) The effect of Trendelenburg tilt and other procedures on the position of endotracheal tubes. *Lancet*, **i**, 850–853

Hirsch, J. (1981) Prevention of deep venous thrombosis. *British Journal of Hospital Medicine*, **25**, 143–147

Hirsch, N. P., Smith, G. B. and Hirsch, P. O. (1986) Alfred Kirstein, pioneer of direct laryngoscopy. *Anaesthesia*, **41**, 42–45

Inglis, J. M. and Brook, B. N. (1956) Trendelenburg tilt: obsolete position. *British Medical Journal*, **2**, 343–344

Jackson, C. (1907) *Tracheobronchoscopy, Esophagoscopy and Gastroscopy*. C. V. Mosby, St Louis

Kirstein A. (1886) Autoskopie des larynx und der trachea. *Berliner Klinischer Wochenschrift*, **22**, 476–478

Lincoln, J. R. and Sawyer, H. P. (1961) Complications related to body positions during surgical procedures. *Anesthesiology*, **22**, 800–809

Lyons, G. (1985) Failed intubation. Six years' experience in a teaching maternity unit. *Anaesthesia*, **40**, 759–762

Martin, J. T. (1978) *Positioning in Anaesthesia and Surgery*, pp. 5–7. W. B. Saunders Co., Philadelphia, London, Toronto

Meyer, W. (1885) Trendelenburg's elevated position. *Archiv für Klinische Chirurgie*, **31**, 494

O'Donovan, N., Healy, T. E. J., Faragher, E. B., Wilkins, R. E. and Hamilton, A. A. (1986) Postoperative backache: the use of an inflatable wedge. *British Journal of Anaesthesia*, **58**, 280–283

Sellick, B. A. (1961) Cricoid pressure to control regurgitation of stomach contents during induction of anaesthesia. *Lancet*, **ii**, 404–406

Swain, J. (1960) The case for abandoning the Trendelenburg position in pelvic surgery. *Medical Journal of Australia*, **ii**, 536–537

Trendelenburg, F. (1890) *Sammlung Klinischer Vortrage*, p. 3373. Volkmanns, Leipzig

Utting, J. E., Gray, T. C. and Shelley, F. C. (1979) Human misadventure in anaesthesia. *Canadian Anaesthetists Society Journal*, **26**, 472–478

Chapter two

The lithotomy position

This is a modification of the supine position in which the knees and hips are flexed, and the hips abducted to permit surgical access to the perineum. The term is derived from the ancient operation of 'cutting for stone' (Greek: lithotomica) for which this approach was used.

In British hospitals it is common practice for the ankles to be supported in canvas stirrups held by vertical poles attached to each side of the operating table (*Figure 2.1*). As an alternative, the 'Bierhoff' leg holders (*Figure 2.2*) appear to be a satisfactory method (Goldstein, 1978). The various 'straight leg sling systems' have been associated with sciatic and femoral nerve sequelae and cannot therefore be recommended (*Figure 2.3*) (McQuarrie et al., 1972). The lithotomy position is extensively used in the specialties of gynaecology, urology and anorectal surgery and, for the last 50 years, it has become a common position for childbirth in the majority of maternity hospitals. It is often combined with a minor degree of head-down tilt to enhance venous return; steeper degrees of tilt may be requested if laparoscopy is being performed or access to deep pelvic structures is required.

At first sight this position may appear simple and innocuous. Unfortunately this is not the case and the hazards of its use are many and well documented. The following sections are therefore of particular importance.

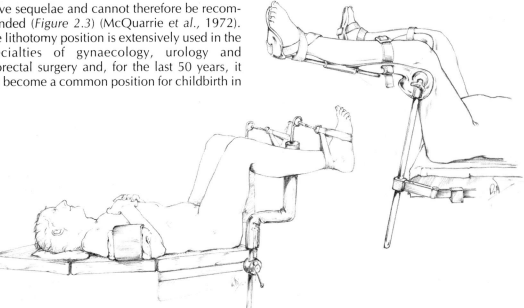

Figure 2.1 The conventional British system for the lithotomy position

Figure 2.2 The Bierhoff system of leg holders commonly used in North America

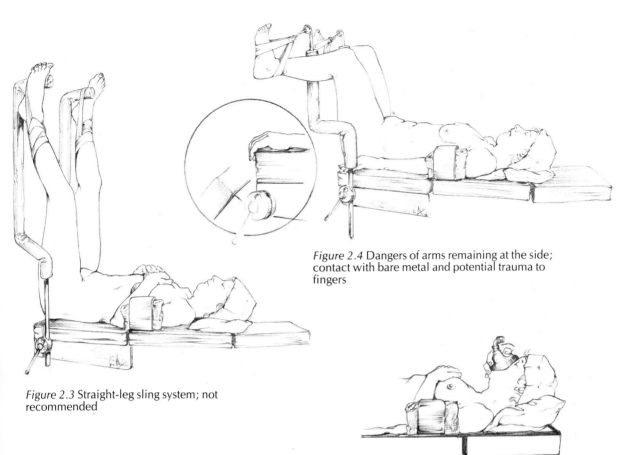

Figure 2.4 Dangers of arms remaining at the side; contact with bare metal and potential trauma to fingers

Figure 2.3 Straight-leg sling system; not recommended

Anatomical hazards

(1) Risks to structures of the face and brachial plexus are as previously described. The arms should be positioned across the patient's chest, wherever possible. If they are allowed to remain by the patient's side, the fingers may overlap the bottom of the table. Ease of metal contact puts them at risk from diathermy burns and manipulation of the bottom section of the operating table can result in the amputation of digits (Courington and Little, 1968) (*Figure 2.4*). Ease of venous access is a secondary but important advantage when the arms are folded across the chest but it may be preferable to have one arm on a board for other reasons, such as invasive monitoring.

(2) Following induction of anaesthesia the patient is moved down the table and the legs are raised up and secured in position. The potential for musculoskeletal strain or damage is as follows:

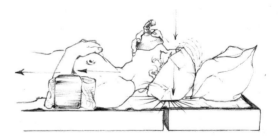

Figure 2.5 Risk to neck resulting from failure to move head support with the patient

(a) the cervical spine is at risk when the patient is moved down the table and it should always be supported on a pillow by the anaesthetist (*Figure 2.5*). Damage is rare but patients with degenerative or rheumatic disease in this region are always at risk from this manoeuvre.

(b) The hips, knees and back are at risk simply because, under general anaesthesia with, or even without, use of muscle relaxants, a range of movement may be attempted which would not be feasible in the conscious patient. It is, therefore, vital to take a proper history from the patient relating to problems with these areas and where necessary, to test the range of permissible movement prior to anaesthesia. Force must never be used and both lower limbs must be moved synchronously. Although backache occurs in up to one-third of postoperative lithotomy patients, this is of comparable frequency to that found in supine patients. The incidence increases with the duration of surgery (Brown and Elman, 1961). Flexion of the hip causes loss of the normal lumbar lordosis. The use of an inflatable wedge to support the lumbosacral curve has been shown to reduce this significantly (O'Donovan et al., 1986). However, it will not ameliorate sacro-iliac or hip joint strains caused by poor positioning technique. In theory at least, acute exacerbation of prolapsed intervertebral disc is a distinct possibility as a result of the forward flexion of the lumbar spine (*Figure 2.6*). Problems with limited mobility of the knees are generally easier to accommodate by altering the inclination of the stirrup supports (*Figure 2.7*); great care must be taken not to force them into unaccustomed positions. In extreme disease the legs may simply be separated and supported on a double arm-board (*Figure 2.8*).

Figure 2.6 Posterior intervertebral disc protrusion resulting from forward flexion of the lumbar spine

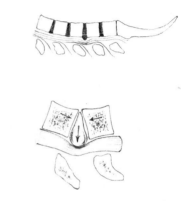

Figure 2.7 Modified lithotomy position for patients with restricted joint movement

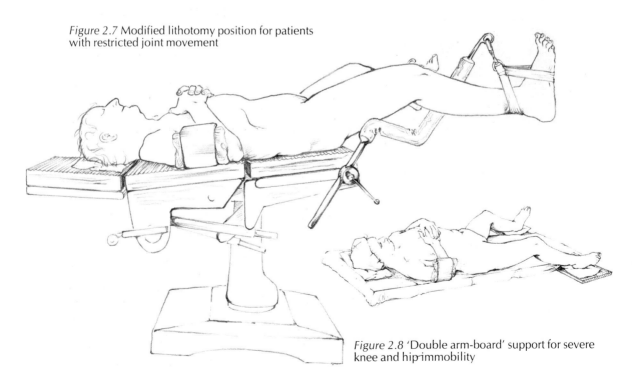

Figure 2.8 'Double arm-board' support for severe knee and hip immobility

(3) Lower limb nerves particularly at risk

(a) The sciatic nerve

Sunderland (1953) has drawn attention to the fact that the sciatic nerve is relatively fixed to underlying structures both at the sciatic notch in the pelvis, and where its common peroneal branch passes around the neck of the fibula. It is important to place the legs in a position that will minimize stretching between these two points (*Figure 2.9*). Variations of the lithotomy position in which the legs were held fully extended and almost vertical to the body have been associated with (reversible) sciatic nerve damage (Burkhardt and Daly, 1966; McQuarrie *et al.*, 1972) (*see Figure 2.3*). They should therefore be avoided. External rotation of the hip with the legs in the more conventional lithotomy position again puts the sciatic nerve at risk. Surgical assistants should be discouraged from leaning against the knees and thus exerting any pressure which might produce such stretching (Burkhart and Daly, 1966). It has also been postulated that in a small minority of patients damage to the sciatic nerve might result from direct compression of its vascular supply at the sciatic notch (Romfh and Currier, 1983). If this is the case, it is difficult to see why there is not more extensive evidence of ischaemia, since the artery concerned is said to be a major arterial source for the lower limb. Intramuscular injections into the gluteal region should not be given whilst the patient is in the lithotomy position. The sciatic nerve becomes displaced laterally, is more superficial, and hence at greater risk of direct trauma from the needle or the contents of the syringe.

(b) The posterior tibial nerve may theoretically be injured when Bierhoff type stirrups are used to support the posterior aspects of the knee. Undue weight on the popliteal fossa may cause compression of the nerve (Costley, 1972). There do not appear to be any clinical reports to support this contention.

(c) The common peroneal nerve may be compressed against the head of the fibula. As previously stated, flexion of the hip and knees results in stretching of the sciatic nerve, and minor degrees of external pressure are therefore likely to cause damage (Britt and Gordon, 1964). Surgical assistants must not lean directly against the knees when the legs are placed outside the lithotomy poles (*Figure 2.10*), and the nerve should be protected by extra padding if the legs are placed inside the poles (*Figure 2.11*).

(d) The saphenous nerve may be compressed against the medial tibial condyle if the legs are placed outside the vertical stirrup support. Again adequate padding must be provided (*Figure 2.12*).

(e) The obturator nerve may, in theory, be stretched by flexion at the foramen where it leaves the pelvis to enter the thigh. However, since the proximal part of the nerve has an intrapelvic course, it is much more likely to be damaged surgically or by obstetric manipulation.

(f) The femoral nerve can be damaged by being kinked around the tough inguinal ligament (*Figure 2.13*). This complication has been described in association with the use of straight-rod leg supports with swing stirrups (*see Figure 2.3*). These allowed extreme adduction of the thighs with external rotation of the hip (Roblee, 1967; Tondare *et al.*,

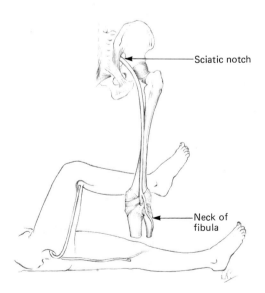

Sciatic notch

Neck of fibula

Figure 2.9 Anatomical fixation of sciatic nerve may predispose to damage from tension

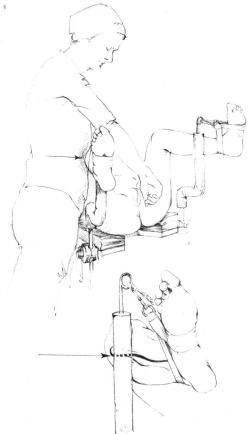

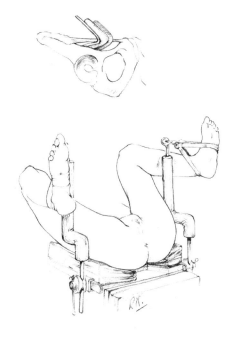

Figure 2.13 Potential damage to the femoral neurovascular bundle from kinking around the inguinal ligament due to extreme flexion, adduction and external rotation of the thighs

Figure 2.10 (upper) Surgical assistant must avoid compressing the patient's leg against the lithotomy support
Figure 2.11 (lower) Potential damage to the common peroneal nerve if leg is positioned inside lithotomy support

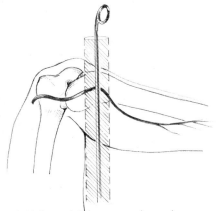

Figure 2.12 Potential damage to the saphenous nerve and vein if the leg is positioned outside the lithotomy support

1983). It is worth noting that the self-retaining abdominal retractors commonly used in pelvic surgery have been incriminated as a cause of femoral nerve damage (Kinges, Wilbanks and Cole, 1965). This knowledge may be of value when blame for such an injury is being apportioned.

(4) Compression and damage to the calf veins is probably the commonest and most dangerous anatomical hazard of the lithotomy position. The stirrup supports should be enclosed completely in foam padding along their entire length and they should be positioned so that there is little or no pressure on the adjacent leg (Figure 2.14). This, however, is often a counsel of perfection and it may be impossible to avoid some compression of the long saphenous veins against the lateral aspect of the stirrups. Blood flow from the calves should be encouraged by

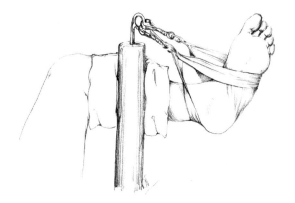

Figure 2.14 Protective pad

correct positioning and, in long operations, the use of external compression apparatus or electrical stimulation gaiters should be considered to reduce the incidence of postoperative deep venous thrombosis. Elastic stockings are also sometimes similarly used. Surgical and nursing assistants must not be allowed to lean against the thighs and legs.

Any direct external pressure on the muscles of the anterolateral aspect of the leg can lead to oedema and swelling. This is called the 'compartment syndrome'. Since these muscles are enclosed within a well defined fascial sheath, there is a risk that the arterial blood supply will become compromised. This, in turn, will lead to further ischaemia and oedema formation. Postoperatively, the legs will be found to be very painful and tender. The early stages can mimic deep venous thrombosis, and it is important that the correct diagnosis is made. The only reliable method of terminating the ischaemia–oedema cycle is for surgical decompression (i.e. fasciotomy) to be expeditiously performed. There are two reports in the literature of compartment syndrome occurring in patients having prolonged surgery in the lithotomy position (Leff and Shapiro, 1979; Lydon and Spielman, 1984). It may be of significance that in both cases the leg support system involved pressure below the popliteal fossa. The dangers of failing to diagnose and treat the condition are postoperative renal failure and permanent loss of function in the muscles affected.

Other hazards of the lithotomy position

(1) Hazards from diathermy apparatus are probably increased in patients placed in the lithotomy position. The earth electrode should always be placed on the thigh and well away from possible contact with fluids used for either skin preparation or urological irrigation. Application of the electrode should be delayed until after the legs have been placed in the stirrups in order to ensure that good skin contact is not lost. A reduction in thigh circumference can be a consequence of the venous drainage associated with change in position. Intraoperative change in patient position should always be accompanied by removal and re-application of the diathermy electrode to ensure that good skin contact is retained.

(2) Induction of general anaesthesia with the patient already in the lithotomy position is only likely to be requested in emergency situations associated with difficulties of childbirth. The combination of flexed thighs and enlarged gravid uterus cause a marked rise in intra-abdominal pressure and make regurgitation of gastric contents a serious and unacceptable risk (Spence, Moir and Finlay, 1967). Furthermore, the fixed supine position makes clearance of mouth and pharynx much more difficult than when the patient can be turned rapidly into the lateral position. This is even more pertinent when it is considered that the head-down tilt mechanism on many makes of labour ward bed is not easily accessible and is inefficient in operation. It is therefore essential that, even in cases of extreme urgency, general anaesthesia should never be induced with the patient in the lithotomy position. The legs should be removed temporarily from the stirrups, straightened and held by assistants ready for replacement as soon as induction and security of the airway have been achieved (Moir, 1980). The presence of other assistants who could tilt the table or assist with turning the patient laterally is mandatory.

Induction of anaesthesia in non-pregnant patients in the lithotomy position is only very rarely required and the anaesthetist will have to judge each case individually, bearing in mind the foregoing comments.

(3) Failure to fasten the stirrup straps correctly or to tighten the stirrup supports properly is a

very real and worrying risk. Pressure from assistants may then just be sufficient to cause the leg to fall whilst the other side remains fixed. Severe back strain or damage to the hip and knee joints could ensue, particularly in the elderly or arthritic patient.

(4) Where significant surgical bleeding occurs the lithotomy position can engender a false sense of security for the anaesthetist. Auto-transfusion from the venous sinuses of the calf and leg muscles will mask the true extent of the blood volume deficit. When the legs are lowered at the completion of surgery between 500 and 800 ml of blood may be drained back into the lower extremities, depending on the depth of anaesthesia and the degree of vasodilatation (Little, 1960). This sudden loss of circulating blood volume can cause marked hypotension and particularly jeopardize the poor-risk patient. Much of the danger can be reduced or even eliminated by slow, gentle and smooth movement of the patient. The assistants, therefore, must be careful and unhurried at this stage of the proceedings, and further transfer from the operating table must be delayed until the anaesthetist is totally sure that the cardiovascular state is stable and satisfactory.

Preliminary anaesthetic considerations

Routine induction of anaesthesia is performed in the supine position. A double-length of breathing hose from the anaesthetic machine allows movement of the patient down the table without the necessity to disconnect, move the anaesthetic machine or risk extubating the patient inadvertently.

Operating table

With the standard general-surgical type of operating table it is necessary to move the patient down towards lithotomy poles situated at the foot-end of the table. In recent years this problem has been overcome by the development of tables on which the legs can be placed in the lithotomy position; the complete lower half of the operating table then folds away and the upper section supporting the patient slides, on rails, to the foot-end of the table.

Positioning the patient (general-surgical operating table)

(1) The arms should be secured across the patient's chest. If 'arm retainers' are used they should be inserted directly under the patient, and not beneath the stretcher canvas or mattress. In this way, they remain *in situ* and prevent the arms from falling off the side of the operating table when the patient is moved (*Figure 2.15*).

(2) Next, the stirrups are positioned on each side to the surgeon's requirements ensuring that they are completely symmetrical.

(3) A minimum of two assistants is required. They must be fully briefed. The anaesthetist takes responsibility for the head and neck.

(4) One assistant lifts the patient's pelvis sufficiently clear of the table for a foam pad or inflatable support to be inserted beneath the lumbar curvature of the spine (*Figure 2.16*).

(5) The first assistant is then positioned at the foot of the patient and the second assistant at one side, level with the patient's hips.

(6) The two assistants then pull the stretcher canvas down the table until the hips are level with the stirrup supports. At no time must the patient's calves be permitted to rest on the end of the operating table (*Figures 2.17* and *2.18*).

(7) The legs are then lifted *together* and the ankles placed in the canvas supports or slings (*Figures 2.19, 2.20* and *2.21*). Adjustment may be needed to ensure a central position, and the placing of the lumbar support should be checked. Depending on the model of operating table, the bottom third is then either folded down or removed completely. Some gynaecologists who use a dependent type of vaginal speculum prefer the perineum to be over the lower edge of the table.

Implicit during the whole procedure is the basic principle that at no time must any force be used. If there is resistance, it may be due to organic disease (arthritis, etc) or insufficient anaesthesia. Both must be judged by the anaesthetist. If there is pre-existing joint disease or deformity, a modified position may have to be agreed with the surgeon beforehand.

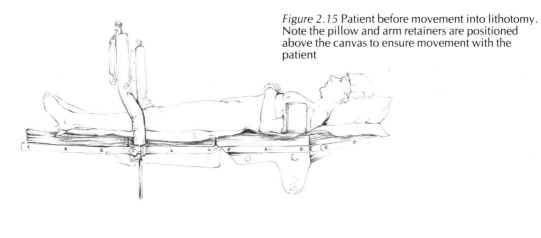

Figure 2.15 Patient before movement into lithotomy. Note the pillow and arm retainers are positioned above the canvas to ensure movement with the patient

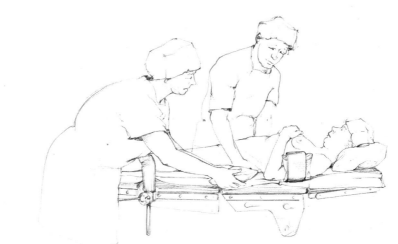

Figure 2.16 Insertion of lumbosacral support

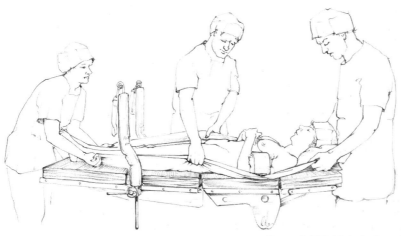

Figure 2.17 Initial placing of positioning team

24

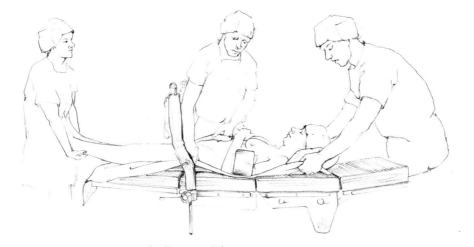

Figure 2.18 Hips positioned adjacent to lithotomy supports

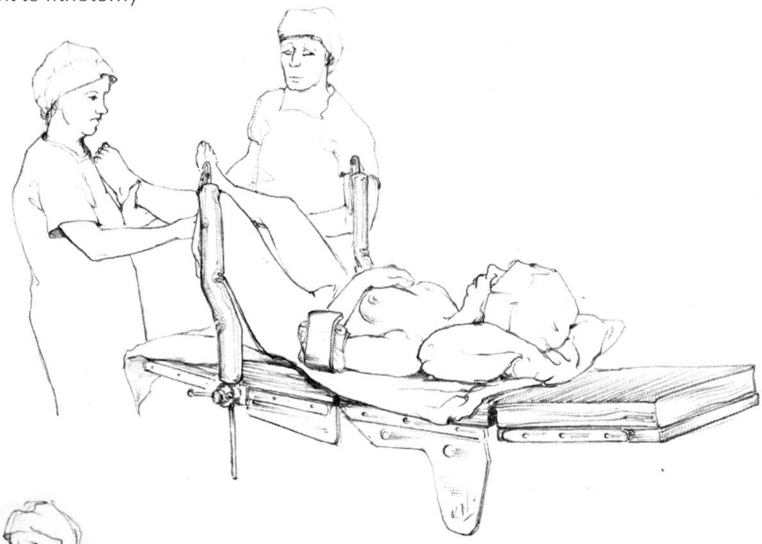

Figure 2.19 Simultaneous lifting of legs

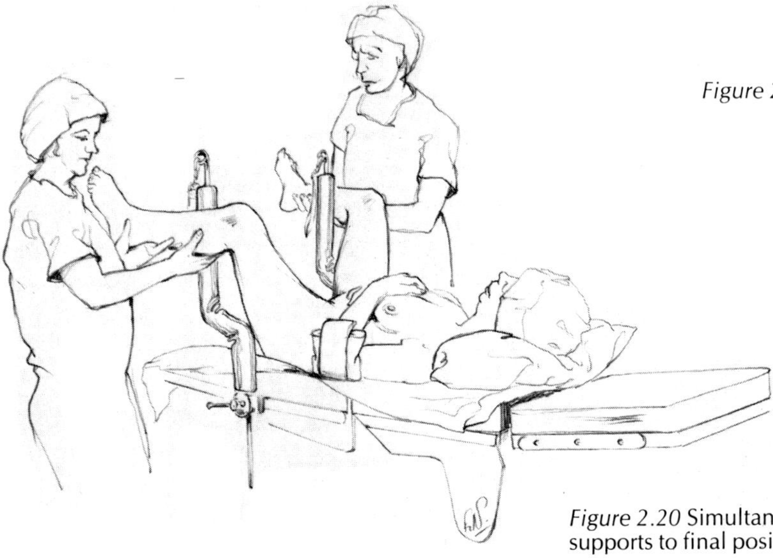

Figure 2.20 Simultaneous elevation of legs over the supports to final position

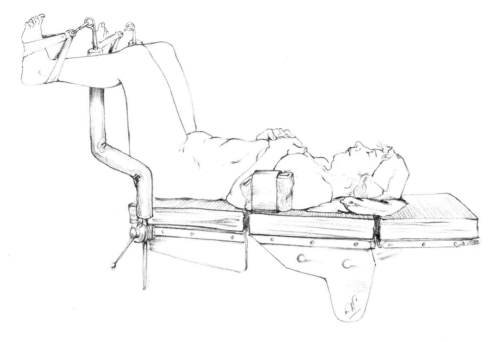

Figure 2.21 Final position with feet in stirrups

Return to the recovery position

The potential for producing musculoskeletal damage is just as great when taking the patient down from lithotomy as at the beginning. Vigilance at this stage is mandatory.

(1) The lower end of the operating table is first replaced in the horizontal position or lifted as appropriate.

(2) The anaesthetist must check that the breathing hoses are free to follow when the patient is moved.

(3) With an attendant on either side of the operating table, the patient is moved back with both legs still supported in the stirrups until the knees are partly deflexed.

(4) The feet are then both removed from the stirrups *together* and the patient is moved the remainder of the distance up the operating table.

(5) Only when the legs and ankles can rest completely on the table should the legs be placed in the horizontal position. Both sides must be moved simultaneously.

Positioning the patient (special operating tables)

(1) The patient is placed on the operating table with the hips at the level of the lithotomy poles.

(2) Following induction of anaesthesia the legs are placed on the poles in the manner previously described and the lower half of the mattress is removed (*Figure 2.22*).

(3) The lower section of the table is retracted (*Figure 2.23*).

(4) Patient and upper table section are simultaneously moved to the foot-end of the operating table (*Figure 2.24*).

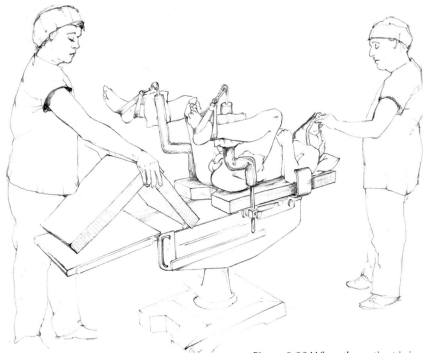

Figure 2.22 When the patient is in position the lower half of the mattress is removed

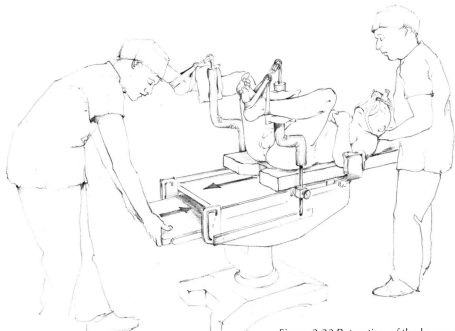

Figure 2.23 Retraction of the lower end of the operating table and movement of the upper section and patient

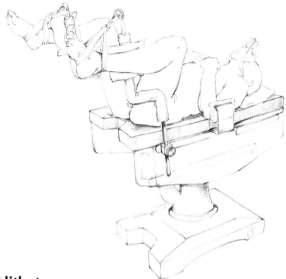

Figure 2.24 The final position

Variations of the standard lithotomy position

Modified lithotomy with Trendelenburg

The standard lithotomy stirrups are used but with less flexion of the thighs in order to allow better surgical access to the abdomen. A varying amount of tilt is required when vaginal manipulations are accompanied by laparoscopic examination of the pelvic organs (*Figure 2.25*). Gravitational displacement of the bowel away from the latter permits a better operative view. If laparoscopic diathermy procedures are performed it is important not to level the patient until sufficient time has elapsed for the tissues to cool adequately; adhesions to the bowel should not then occur. Levelling before the gas has been vented may cause it to accumulate under the diaphragm with consequent postoperative discomfort.

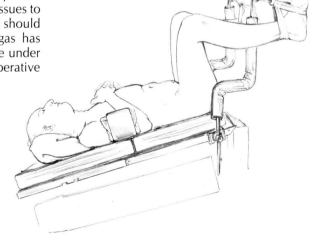

Figure 2.25 Combined lithotomy and Trendelenburg position

The Lloyd Davies position (originally called the lithotomy–Trendelenburg position)

This is used where any combined perineal and abdominal surgical approach is required. Abdominoperineal resection of the rectum is the classic procedure performed in this position. As will be seen from the illustration (*Figure 2.26*), the multijointed leg supports offer a wide range of adjustment and allow for much less flexion of the hips and knees (Lloyd Davies, 1939). The calves are supported directly by semicylindrical padded rests. The legs should be lightly bandaged into the latter to prevent displacement by surgical assistants. Access to the perineum is secured more by abducting the thighs than by flexing them and is enhanced by placing a firm pad beneath the sacrum so that the sacrococcygeal articulation projects some 2.5–3.0 cm beyond its distal edge (*Figure 2.27*). The fact that the hips are not so flexed as in the conventional lithotomy position permits the abdominal surgeon, and his assistant on the opposite side of the table, adequate access to the pelvis. There can be some conflict of interest between the anaesthetists and the theatre nursing team who are competing for the remaining available space around the head-end of the operating table. These operations are often accompanied by serious blood loss and it is essential that the patient's arms should be arranged so that the anaesthetist has impeccable access for both monitoring the peripheral circulation and administering intravenous fluids. Surgical texts (Goligher, 1984; Thorlakson, 1984) on this subject depict instrument tables placed over the patient's head and the patient's arms placed alongside the body. In the authors' experience both these factors can leave the anaesthetist dangerously remote from the patient. Amicable discussion with the nursing staff over the siting of their equipment has resulted in the compromise that overhead instrument tables are no longer used, providing that the anaesthetist does not encroach on the left-hand, head-end side of the patient. If necessary the right arm may be placed out laterally on a board, otherwise both arms are supported across the chest below the screen (*Figure 2.28*). Operating table and instrument trolleys are sited as in the illustration (*Figure 2.29*).

Finally the table is tipped into approximately 20 degrees of Trendelenburg tilt; greater degrees of tilt should not be required and, with modern operating table non-slip mattresses, there is no requirement for dangerous shoulder supports. The latter have, in the past, been responsible for at least one successful medicolegal claim for negligence after causing brachial plexus nerve damage (MedicoLegal Abstracts, 1945).

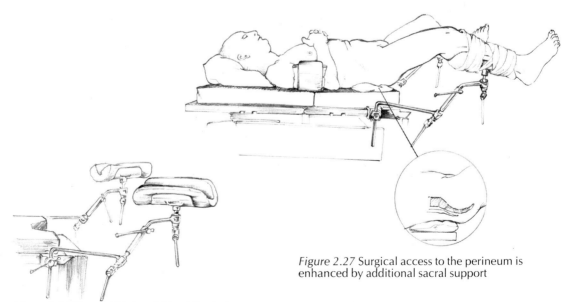

Figure 2.27 Surgical access to the perineum is enhanced by additional sacral support

Figure 2.26 The multi-jointed 'Lloyd Davies' supports

Extremes of lithotomy

These positions, in which the thighs were flexed back almost adjacent to the abdominal wall, should no longer be necessary. Although previously in vogue for some pelvic procedures and perineal prostatectomy, modern anaesthetic and surgical techniques have made the position obsolete. The obvious dangers to the sciatic, femoral and obturator nerves have been dealt with earlier in the chapter.

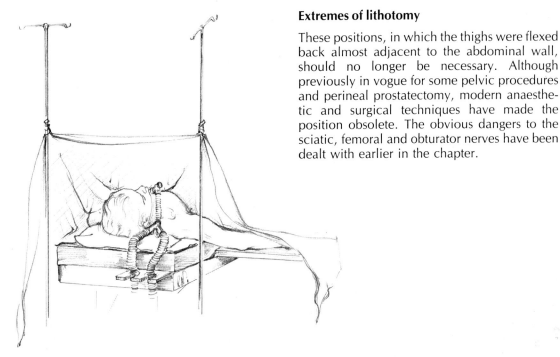

Figure 2.28 Screen shielding anaesthetic area from surgical site

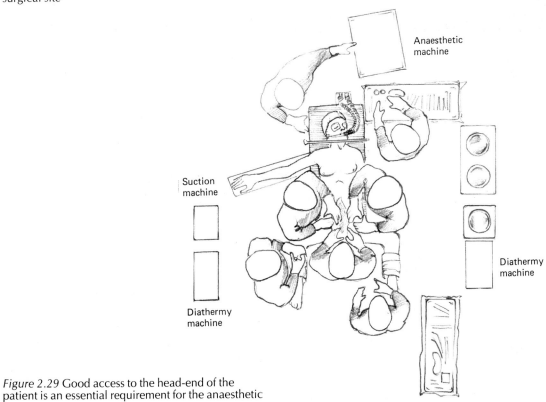

Figure 2.29 Good access to the head-end of the patient is an essential requirement for the anaesthetic

References

Britt, B. A. and Gordon, R. A. (1964) Peripheral nerve injuries associated with anaesthesia. *Canadian Anaesthetists Society Journal,* **2**, 514–535

Brown, E. M. and Elman, D. S. (1961) Postoperative backache. *Anesthesia and Analgesia,* **40**, 683–685

Burkhart, F. L. and Daly, J. W. (1966) Sciatic and peroneal nerve injury. A complication of vaginal operations. *Obstetrics and Gynecology,* **28**, 99–102

Costley, D. O. (1972) Peripheral nerve injury. *International Anaesthesiology Clinics,* **10** (Spring volume) (No. 1), 189–206

Courington, F. W. and Little, D. M. (1968) Clinical anaesthesia 3: The role of posture in anaesthesia. In *Common and Uncommon Problems in Anesthesiology,* pp. 24–54. Edited by M. T. Jenlans. F. A. Davis Co., Philadelphia

Goldstein, P. J. (1978) The lithotomy position. In *Positioning in Anesthesia and Surgery,* pp. 142–161. Edited by J. T. Martin. W. B. Saunders, Philadelphia

Goligher, J. (1984) *Surgery of the Anus, Rectum and Colon,* 5th edn, pp. 620–621. Balliere Tindall, London

Kinges, K. G., Wilbanks, G. D. and Cole, G. R. (1965) Injury to the femoral nerve during pelvic operations. *Obstetrics and Gynecology,* **25**, 619–623

Leff, R. G. and Shapiro, S. R. (1979) Lower extremity complications of the lithotomy position. Prevention and management. *Journal of Urology,* **122**, 138–139

Little, D. M. Jnr. (1960) Posture and anaesthesia. *Canadian Anaesthetists Society Journal,* **7**, 2–15

Lloyd Davies, O. V. (1939) Lithotomy–Trendelenburg position for resection of the rectum and lower pelvic colon. *Lancet,* **ii**, 74–76

Lydon, J. C. and Spielman, F. J. (1984) Bilateral compartment syndrome following prolonged surgery in the lithotomy position. *Anesthesiology,* **60**, 236–238

McQuarrie, H. G., Harris, S. W., Ellsworth, H. S., Stone, R. D. and Anderson, A. E. (1972) Sciatic neuropathy complicating vaginal hysterectomy. *American Journal of Obstetrics and Gynecology,* **113**, 223–232

MedicoLegal Abstracts (1945) Malpractice: Injury to the anaesthetized patient. *Journal of the American Medical Association,* **127**, 734–735

Moir, D. D. (1980) *Obstetric Anaesthesia and Analgesia,* 2nd edn, p. 154. Balliere Tindall, London

O'Donovan, N., Healy, T. E. J., Farragher, E. B., Wilkins, R. G. and Hamilton, A. A. (1986) Postoperative backache: the use of an inflatable wedge. *British Journal of Anaesthesia,* **58**, 280–283

Roblee, M. A. (1967) Femoral neuropathy from the lithotomy position. Case report and a new leg holder for prevention. *American Journal of Obstetrics and Gynecology,* **97**, 871–872

Romfh, J. H. and Currier, R. D. (1983) Sciatic neuropathy induced by the lithotomy position. *Archives of Neurology,* **40**, 127

Spence, A. A., Moir, D. D. and Finlay, W. E. I. (1967) Observations on intragastric pressure. *Anaesthesia,* **22**, 249–255

Sunderland, S. (1953) Relative susceptibility to injury of the medial and lateral divisions of the sciatic nerve. *British Journal of Surgery,* **41**, 300–302

Thorlakson, R. H. (1984) A simplified draping of patients in the lithotomy–Trendelenburg position for anterior resection by stapling or abdominal perineal excision of the rectum. *Diseases of the Colon and Rectum,* **27**, 204–206

Tondare, A. S., Nadkarni, A. V., Sathe, C. H. and Dave, V. B. (1983) Femoral neuropathy: a complication of lithotomy position under spinal anaesthesia. *Canadian Anaesthetists Society Journal,* **30**, 84–86

Chapter three

The lateral position

The majority of surgical operations performed with the patient in the lateral position are complicated and time consuming. This position is used in pulmonary and oesophageal work, renal surgery and some neurosurgical procedures. It is essential with the lateral position to strike a balance between achieving stability of the patient and protection of structures at risk through pressure. Considerable alterations in cardiorespiratory physiology are known to occur and may be exacerbated by the nature of the surgical operation.

Anatomical hazards

(1) Proper support for the head is essential. Necrosis of the underlying ear can be caused by pressure of the head if it is not supported on a soft pillow, or if it is trapped against an inadequately padded 'horseshoe support' (*Figure 3.1*). Specially designed head-rests, which secure the skull position by percutaneous skeletal fixation, are commonly used for this reason in many neurosurgical procedures.

(2) The brachial plexus of the upper arm can be stretched if the head is allowed to be too dependent (*Figure 3.2*). This danger can be compounded if, in the interests of better surgical access, the shoulder and upper arm have skin traction applied to hold them away from the operation site.

(3) The brachial plexus of the dependent arm must always be protected by a pad placed high in the underlying axilla (*Figure 3.3*). This also serves to relieve pressure on the adjacent

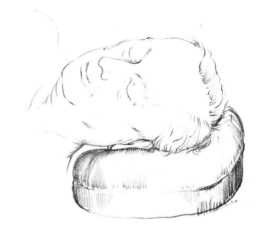

Figure 3.1 Care must be taken to ensure that the ear does not become trapped

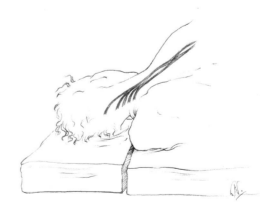

Figure 3.2 The brachial plexus of the upper arm can be stretched if the head is allowed to be too dependent

31

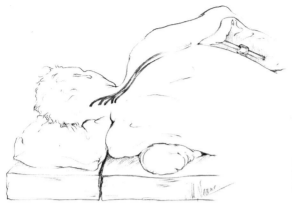

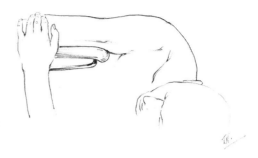

Figure 3.4 The upper arm support should not touch the chest wall. It must not be angled in order to protect the radial nerve

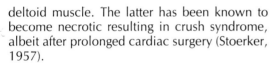

Figure 3.3 The brachial plexus of the lower arm must be protected by a supporting pad under the apex of the axilla. Support of the head relieves potential tension of the upper brachial plexus

deltoid muscle. The latter has been known to become necrotic resulting in crush syndrome, albeit after prolonged cardiac surgery (Stoerker, 1957).

(4) The upper arm is usually supported on a special adjustable arm-rest. This must not be in a position where an edge can compress the radial nerve in the spiral groove of the humerus nor should it press against the skin of the chest wall (*Figure 3.4*). The ulnar nerve at the elbow is unlikely to be at risk unless it is abnormally superficial.

(5) The skin over the lower iliac crest is particularly at risk from pressure necrosis in long operations. In these it is wise to position the patient on a soft sheepskin rug. An alternative that has recently become available is the evacuatable mattress (*see* Chapter 7). This effectively spreads the weight-load of the patient evenly.

(6) Very rarely, in emaciated patients placed in the lateral position, the underlying sciatic nerve can be damaged by direct pressure on the buttock at the point where it exits from the pelvis (Parks, 1973).

Bony prominences of the lower limbs are obviously at risk and should be correctly supported by pillows (*Figure 3.5*). The use of external pneumatic compression apparatus will give useful protection by rhythmically separat-

ing the legs. The common peroneal nerve, as it winds round the neck of the fibula, is particularly vulnerable.

Preliminary anaesthetic considerations

(1) The basic requirements for induction of anaesthesia have been covered in the previous chapters and need not be reiterated. It is worthwhile re-checking that all the necessary ancillary apparatus for keeping the patient in position is available and in working order. This will prevent unnecessary delays occurring after the patient has been anaesthetized.

(2) Induction of general anaesthesia and endotracheal intubation is usually carried out with the patient in the supine position, but very occasionally this may be necessary with the patient fully lateral. It has been advocated as a safer alternative in patients with a full stomach, or for Caesarean section patients (Parry Brown, 1973; Latimer and Pearce, 1984) but in neither case has the technique been widely accepted. If it is necessary, precautions must be taken to ensure that adequate support will prevent undue body or limb movement following loss of consciousness. It must also be remembered that intubation will generally be much easier in the left lateral position as the tongue will fall naturally under the bevel of the McIntosh laryngoscope.

(3) Intravenous infusions and arterial monitoring cannulae should preferably be sited in the uppermost arm both for ease of access and reduced likelihood of obstruction.

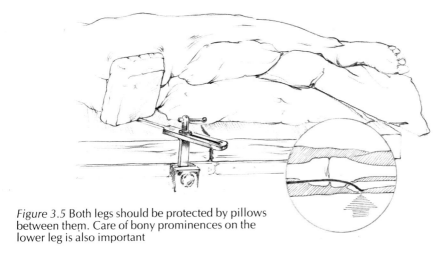

Figure 3.5 Both legs should be protected by pillows between them. Care of bony prominences on the lower leg is also important

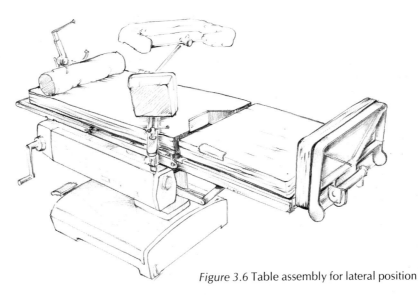

Figure 3.6 Table assembly for lateral position

(4) In thoracic surgical cases one of the specialized double lumen endotracheal tubes will probably be required. In other cases a non-kinkable endotracheal tube should be used. Care in accurate positioning and attention to security are essential to minimize dislodgement when the patient is turned to the lateral position. Access for endotracheal aspiration is easier if the endotracheal tube is positioned at the uppermost angle of the mouth.

(5) A urinary catheter, if required, should be inserted whilst the patient is still in the supine position.

The basic lateral position

Following completion of the anaesthetic induction, the patient is ready to be positioned. It is wise to recheck that all the ancillary table attachments and pillows are at hand and to make sure that the patient is correctly positioned in relation to the break-point of the table (*Figure 3.6*). For most operations, this should be just caudal to the lower margin of the rib cage. The anaesthetist is responsible for care and attention to the head and neck, and coordinates the team of assistants.

Positioning of the assistants

There must be a minimum of two strong assistants and a third to take care of the legs. All assistants should be on the same side of the patient and should be positioned so that during the turning procedure they are rotating the patient away from themselves, i.e. if the patient is to be in the left lateral position, they will stand on the right side of the patient.

(1) The first assistant is positioned to support and turn the patient's chest.

(2) The second assistant supports and turns the pelvis.

(3) The third assistant supports and turns the legs (*Figure 3.7*).

Steps in turning the patient

(1) Check that the operating table brakes are on. The anaesthetist supports the head and neck.

(2) The assistants lift and rotate the patient away from themselves so that the full lateral position is achieved with the patient on the side of the table adjacent to themselves (*Figure 3.8*).

(3) A pillow is placed under the patient's head and the anaesthetic breathing hoses are temporarily secured.

(4) The next step is to insert a firm rubber pad or inflated air cushion into the underlying axilla (*Figure 3.9*). This is done by one assistant whilst the anaesthetist and the 'chest' assistant hold the patient slightly off the surface of the operating table.

(5) With one assistant remaining in position to stabilize the pelvis and chest, the second assistant:
(a) fixes the upper arm on its special adjustable support. The lower arm can be flexed at the elbow and secured with adhesive tape against the side of this arm-rest (*Figure 3.10*) or placed on an arm-board.

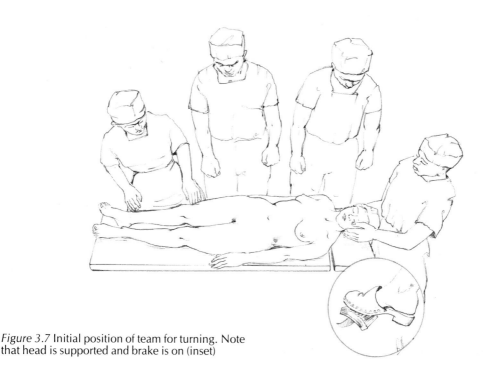

Figure 3.7 Initial position of team for turning. Note that head is supported and brake is on (inset)

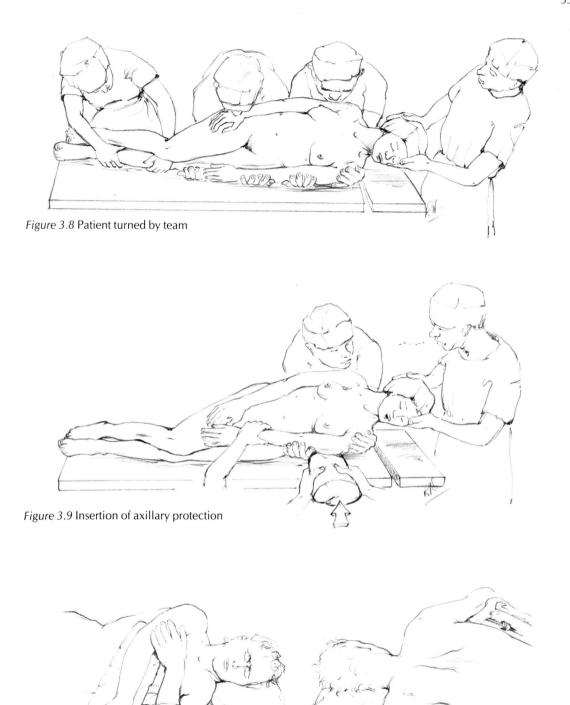

Figure 3.8 Patient turned by team

Figure 3.9 Insertion of axillary protection

Figure 3.10 Placing of arms in lateral position. Inset, position of axillary pad from behind

(b) flexes the patient's thighs and inserts the 'seat support' against the ischial tuberosities (*Figure 3.11*). If this is not possible for any reason a strap placed across the hips may have to suffice.

(6) Attention can now be paid to the lower limbs. Firstly, the diathermy electrode is applied around the uppermost thigh and external compression apparatus is applied to both legs. Pillows are then used to pad and support the semi-flexed limbs, especially between the knees and ankles. The feet are firmly supported against the vertical foot-rest of the table,

particularly if a head-up tilt may be required (*Figure 3.12*).

(7) Finally a strap is secured around the upper pelvic crest and below the operating table. This should not be too tight, but must be capable of preventing the patient from rolling forward under pressure from the surgeon or operating assistants. A pad should be placed between the patient's skin and the strap.

(8) A screen is then placed across the head-end of the table to ensure that the anaesthetist has good access when the surgical drapes have been applied (*Figure 3.13*).

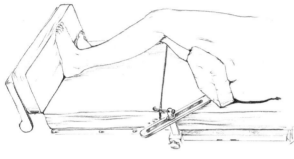

Figure 3.11 Support of buttocks and feet

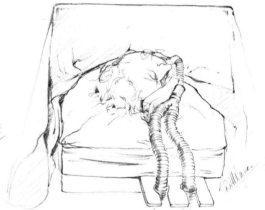

Figure 3.13 Correct position of screen ensures good view and access to anaesthetic assembly

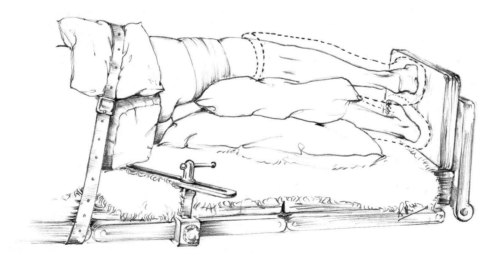

Figure 3.12 Position of legs showing protection by pillows and EPC, feet firmly against vertical foot-rest

Special considerations for neurosurgery in the lateral position

(1) In the pioneer days of neurosurgery it was logical that access to the cervical spine and posterior cranial fossae should be sought with the patient in the sitting position. It gave an excellent view of the surgical field and provided natural drainage for blood, cerebrospinal fluid and irrigation fluids. Unfortunately, the ever-present threat of venous air embolism and potential problems with arterial hypotension have led some centres to completely abandon this position in favour of the prone or full lateral position. A recent survey in the United Kingdom has shown that for surgery on the posterior cranial fossa approximately half the centres still regularly use the sitting position but for operations on the cervical spine fewer than 30 per cent do so (Campkin, 1981). Experience with neurosurgical procedures in the lateral position has shown that surgical access and drainage of fluids from the operation field are comparable and venous air embolism virtually never happens. There have been no fatalities from air embolism in the authors' hospital since this policy was adopted approximately 30 years ago.

(2) The lateral position also presents a satisfactory alternative to the prone position for lower cervical and thoracic spinal operations (*Figure 3.14*). This is particularly important in pregnant or very obese patients or those with cardiovascular problems who would just not tolerate this position. Furthermore, the anaesthetist has much better access to the patient if problems arise in these difficult patients.

(3) Absolute security of the position of trunk and limbs is essential in neurosurgical patients when the head is fixed in a rigid three-pin head-rest. Any movement of the body after this has been locked can throw a dangerous strain on the cervical spine.

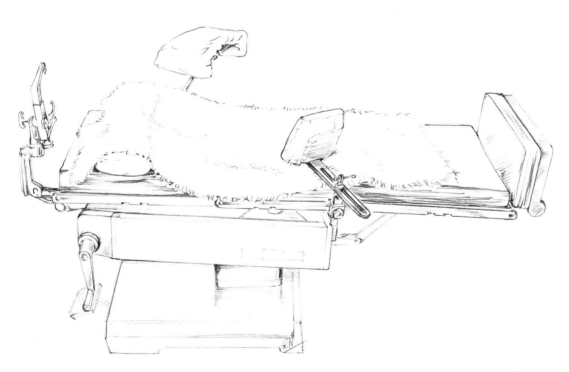

Figure 3.14 Table assembly for lateral position for neurosurgery. Note sheepskin and three-pin head-rest

(4) Surgical access may be improved by the use of broad adhesive strapping to retract the upper shoulder away from the neck (*Figure 3.15*). It can be displaced towards the ipsilateral iliac crest by attaching the strapping over the metal 'seat support'.

(5) The upper shoulder may alternatively be held away from the operating field by lowering it towards the operation table. This is the 'park bench' position (Gilbert, Brindle and Galdino, 1966) (*Figure 3.16*). The lower arm is also placed outstretched on a board. The patient's head is secured in a skull clamp, then elevated, flexed and rotated towards the floor. It is useful for surgery involving the cerebellopontine angle as with acoustic neuromas.

(6) The evacuatable mattress has been mentioned earlier in the chapter as a possible alternative means of support for the laterally positioned patient. It has been found to be particularly acceptable for prolonged neurosurgical procedures. Experience has been gained on patients with operating times in the 8–13

hours range without the occurrence of any postoperative skin pressure problems. It has also been noted that its insulation properties are such that if used in conjunction with an external warming blanket, the patient's temperature will actually rise!

(7) Finally, the reader's attention is drawn to a description in Chapter 5 of the 'lateral sitting position'. This has the great advantage that should resuscitation be necessary the patient is tipped rapidly into the lateral position thus retaining good, sterile access to the operating field.

(8) The very last check to be made after the head has been locked into position and before the surgical skin preparation starts is to ensure that the endotracheal tube has not slipped into the right main bronchus.

Figure 3.16 'Park bench position'

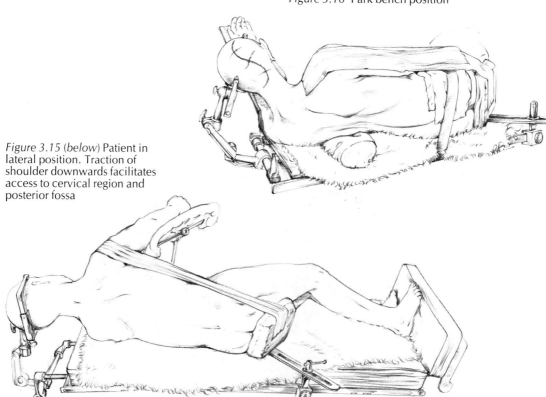

Figure 3.15 (*below*) Patient in lateral position. Traction of shoulder downwards facilitates access to cervical region and posterior fossa

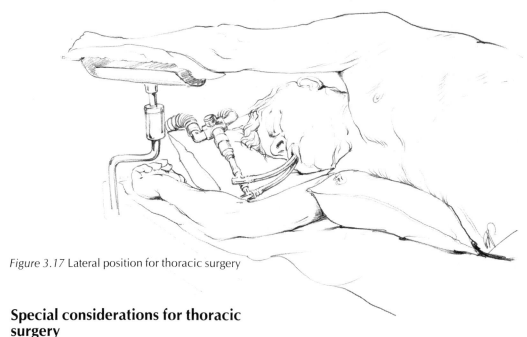

Figure 3.17 Lateral position for thoracic surgery

Special considerations for thoracic surgery

(1) The upper arm support and screen must be arranged so that the anaesthetist has the best possible access to check, manipulate or aspirate the double-lumen endotracheal tube (*Figure 3.17*). The head is usually supported on a soft pillow with the neck in mid-position. Monitoring and infusion lines should allow instant and reliable administration of drugs and fluids.

(2) Improved surgical access may be achieved by the use of an inflatable air cushion beneath the chest (*Figure 3.18*). This helps to spread the intercostal incision and is common practice in many cardiothoracic centres. Tip-ping the bottom half of the table 15 to 20 degrees foot-down can also be of assistance in this respect. The table is straightened and the air cushion deflated to assist in closure of the wound at completion of the operation. Some surgeons prefer the patient to be leaning 10–15 degrees towards them rather than in the full lateral position.

(3) Repositioning the patient at the end of surgery and transfer to the recovery area necessitates an understanding of the management of underwater chest drains and this is dealt with in Chapter 6.

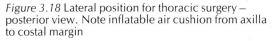

Figure 3.18 Lateral position for thoracic surgery – posterior view. Note inflatable air cushion from axilla to costal margin

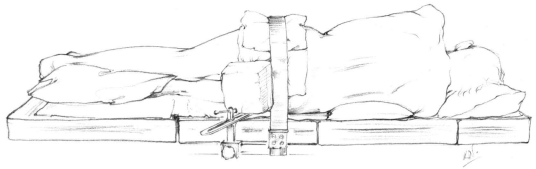

Special considerations for renal and extraperitoneal surgery

(1) The nephrectomy position consists of the patient being placed in the full lateral state but with the operating table broken approximately 20 degrees each way immediately under the flank (*Figure 3.19*). The dependent axilla is supported with a pad and the lower leg is flexed at both the hip and the knee. The use of 'kidney bridges' found on some of the older operating tables has become unnecessary since modern anaesthetic techniques produce excellent muscle relaxation and access for the surgeon. Similarly, the use of the lateral jack-knife position is to be deprecated as it produces marked pooling of blood in both dependent parts of the body. The heart and major vessels may also be distorted and obstructed.

(2) The extra peritoneal approach to the hilum of the liver, the bile ducts and the head of the pancreas can be facilitated by the patient in a semi-lateral position (*Figure 3.20*). Sandbags are inserted under the pelvis and chest on the right-hand side and the table is broken as for a nephrectomy. The patient's right arm is positioned away from the surgical field and across the chest by a special retainer. The other arm is either placed alongside the body or out on a board, if required for access to infusions.

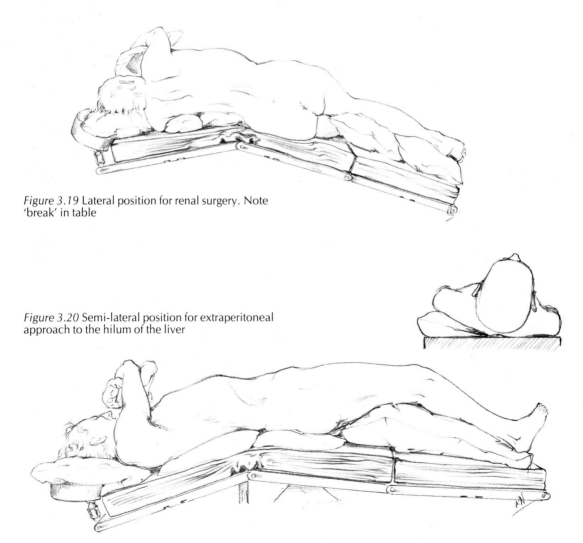

Figure 3.19 Lateral position for renal surgery. Note 'break' in table

Figure 3.20 Semi-lateral position for extraperitoneal approach to the hilum of the liver

Special considerations for the maternity patient

The 'lateral tilt' position

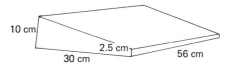

Figure 3.21 'Crawford wedge' for operating theatre use (From Crawford, 1977, with permission of the publishers)

Since the 1970s this position has become standard for any patient requiring surgery in the latter weeks of pregnancy. A foam rubber wedge capable of tipping the patient 10–15 degrees from the horizontal is placed under the right pelvic and flank area (Crawford, 1977) (*Figure 3.21*). Alternatively, a simple inflatable 'wedge' (Carrie, 1982) serves the same function and has the merit that it can be deflated easily following delivery of the infant at Caesarean section. The rationale for this 'lateral tilt' position is based on the fact that a heavy uterus, at or near term, compresses the inferior vena cava when the mother lies fully supine. Credit for first recognizing, investigating and publicizing this observation must go to McRoberts (1951) and Howard, Goodson and Mengert (1953) who described 'postural shock in pregnancy' and 'supine hypotensive syndrome in late pregnancy' respectively. In their patients, the return blood supply to the right side of the heart was so impaired in the supine position that serious falls of blood pressure ensued unless they were allowed to turn onto their sides. Fortunately, the vast majority of pregnant patients do not experience such exaggerated effects due to the fact that they have enlarged paravertebral venous collateral pathways (Kerr, Scott and Samuel, 1964). However, all patients do have some degree of vena cava obstruction with reduced cardiac output (Lees *et al.*, 1967) and in many the aorta is also partly occluded. (Bieniarz, Maqueda and Caldeyro-Barcia, 1966). The adverse circulatory effects are not only confined to the mother as it can be shown that the fetus is delivered in a more satisfactory physiological state when lateral tilt is employed (Crawford, Burton and Davies, 1972). If the vasodilatory and cardiodepressant effects of a general anaesthetic are superimposed on a maternal circulation compromised by aortocaval obstruction the situation can rapidly become life-threatening. It is therefore strongly recommended to use 'lateral tilt' in all cases for surgery at term.

Routine use of this position should never be allowed to engender a sense of false security for the anaesthetist. In the authors' experience even 'a wedge' will not always prevent a serious fall in maternal blood pressure following induction of anaesthesia for Caesarean section. Indeed, it may even delay its onset and allow the maternal cardiovascular system to compensate for a further few minutes. When any such dramatic fall in blood pressure occurs it is vital that there are an adequate number of helpers in the operating theatre to reposition the patient into the full lateral position. If the obstetrician has already opened the peritoneum the crisis can be resolved either by very rapid delivery of the infant or simply by the surgeon holding the gravid uterus forward off the underlying great vessels. Some slight head-down tilt may also be helpful at this time. Once the circulation has been restored for a few minutes the uterus can be replaced and the infant delivered as expeditiously as possible.

If, for any reason, cardiopulmonary resuscitation is required in a pregnant patient near to term, it will be obvious from the foregoing discussion that a successful outcome will be most unlikely if the patient is left in the standard supine position.

Although the above remarks have concentrated on the pregnant patient the cardiovascular disturbances described are equally pertinent to a patient of either sex presenting for surgery with a very large mobile abdominal mass situated above the aorta and inferior vena cava (Schroeder and Jebson, 1986).

References

Bieniarz, J., Maqueda, E. and Caldeyro-Barcia, R. (1966) Compression of the aorta by the uterus in late human pregnancy. *American Journal of Obstetrics and Gynecology*, **95**, 795–807

Campkin, T. V. (1981) Posture and ventilation during posterior fossa and cervical operations. Current practice in the United Kingdom. *British Journal of Anaesthesia*, **53**, 881–883

Carrie, L. E. S. (1982) An inflatable obstetric anaesthetic 'wedge'. *Anaesthesia,* **37**, 745–747

Crawford, J. S., Burton, M. and Davies, P. (1972) Time and lateral tilt at Caesarean section. *British Journal of Anaesthesia,* **44**, 477–484

Crawford, J. S. (1977) *Principles and Practice of Obstetric Anaesthesia,* 4th Edn, p. 245. Blackwell Scientific Publications, Oxford

Gilbert, R. G. B., Brindle, A. F. and Galdino, A. (1966) The park bench position. *Anaesthesia for Neurosurgery,* pp. 119–151. Little Brown & Co., Boston

Howard, B. K., Goodson, J. D. and Mengert, W. F. (1953) Supine hypotensive syndrome in late pregnancy. *Obstetrics and Gynecology,* **i**, 371–377

Kerr, M. G., Scott, D. B. and Samuel, E. (1964) Studies on the inferior vena cava in late pregnancy. *British Medical Journal,* **i**, 532–533

Latimer, R. D. and Pearce, A. J. (1984) Maternal position during induction of anaesthesia for Caesarean section. *Anaesthesia,* **39**, 383

Lees, M. M., Scott, D. B., Kerr, M. G. and Taylor, S. H. (1967) Circulatory effects of supine posture in late pregnancy. *Clinical Science,* **32**, 453–465

McRoberts, W. A. Jnr. (1951) Postural shock in pregnancy. *American Journal of Obstetrics and Gynecology,* **62**, 627–632

Parks, J. B. (1973) Postoperative peripheral neuropathies. *Surgery,* **74**, 348–357

Parry Brown, I. A. (1973) Posture in anaesthesia. *Proceedings of Royal Society of Medicine,* **66**, 339–344

Schroeder, G. M. and Jebson, P. J. (1986) The supine hypotensive syndrome in a young boy. *Anesthesiology,* **64**, 377–378

Stoerker, R. A. (1957) Crush phenomenon. *Anesthesiology,* **18**, 342

Chapter four

The prone position

The prone position is used for surgery on the posterior aspect of the body. Without doubt, it carries a degree of risk greater than any of the positions described in the preceding chapters.

Until the classic paper by Mixter and Barr (1934) relating the symptomatology of sciatic pain to prolapsed intervertebral disc, operations on the vertebral column were relatively rare (Hunter, 1950). Since that time an ever-increasing complexity of surgical procedures on the spinal axis have become commonplace. Coincidentally, varying methods of supporting the patient have evolved. Two important landmarks are worth mentioning.

The first 'frame' for supporting the prone patient was described by Moore and Edmunds in 1950 (*Figure 4.1*), and there have been many others since. The first measurements of inferior vena cava pressure in laminectomy patients were published by Pearce in 1957 (*Figures 4.2* and *4.19*). This established, scientifically, the

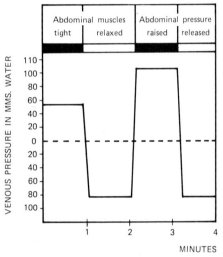

Figure 4.2 Measurements of inferior vena cava pressure in the prone position made by Pearce in 1957 (reproduced by permission of the author and publishers)

Figure 4.1 'Frame' for supporting the prone patient as described by Moore and Edmunds (1950) (reproduced by permission of the author and publishers)

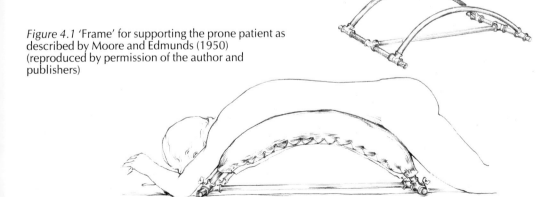

importance of correct positioning and good anaesthesia in minimizing blood loss at the operation site. Haemorrhage due to venous back pressure had, until then, been a formidable obstacle to the surgeon; despite the fact that the wealth of interconnecting channels between the lumbar epidural plexuses and the central venous system had been well documented (Batson, 1940; Norgore, 1945).

Anatomical hazards

From above downwards these are as follows:

(1) The position of the head must be kept as near to normal as possible. Analysis of subjective tests on awake volunteers has shown that any prone posture with the pelvis higher than the chest produces pain in the lower neck and upper back when the patient's head is turned to either side. The back and neck should remain in the same plane and the head in the neutral position wherever possible (Smith, Gramling and Volpitto, 1961).

(2) The face should only be allowed to rest on the forehead and must be properly padded. Pressure on the eyes must not occur under any circumstances. Glaucoma could be precipitated in susceptible patients and blindness resulting from central retinal artery thrombosis has been recorded as a result of pressure from a misplaced horseshoe or Bailey head-rest (Britt and Gordon, 1964) (*Figure 4.3*). Extreme tenderness of the skin of the tip of the nose following prolonged inadvertent pressure has also been observed.

(3) Over-extension of the cervical spine must be avoided at all times, particularly while the patient is being turned and before the chest is properly supported. Cervical cord damage is a possible sequela, especially if the spinal canal is narrowed from osteophytic or disc protrusion. Patients with rheumatoid degeneration are especially at risk.

(4) Abnormal movements of the shoulder joint must not be permitted as dislocation or damage to the joint capsule may occur, and traction injury to the brachial plexus is a remote possibility. Smith, Gramling and Volpitto (1961) have shown that the use of arm-boards was not satisfactory to awake subjects. If the arms were extended on the arm-boards, pain in the shoulders was noted within 10 minutes. If the elbows were flexed and the forearms placed across well-padded arm-boards, the subjects complained of numbness of the hands in 10 to 20 minutes. It is, therefore, preferable that the normal prone sleeping position should be replicated with the arms resting on the table 'above' the head. The humerus must not be allowed to rest over the side of the table with consequent damage to the radial nerve (*Figure 4.4*); the superficial position of the ulnar nerve behind the medial epicondyle must be protected (*Figure 4.5*). For reasons of surgical access, it may be necessary sometimes to position the arms alongside the patient's body, particularly when head and neck surgery is performed (*Figure 4.6*).

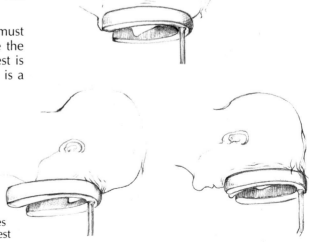

Figure 4.3 The eyes are at risk if the head becomes displaced in either direction on the 'horseshoe' rest

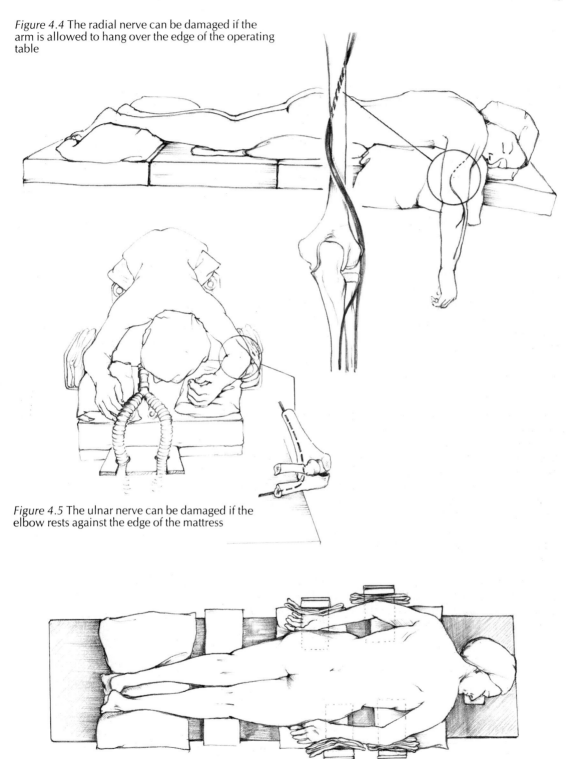

Figure 4.4 The radial nerve can be damaged if the arm is allowed to hang over the edge of the operating table

Figure 4.5 The ulnar nerve can be damaged if the elbow rests against the edge of the mattress

Figure 4.6 Prone position with the arms alongside the body (note position of support pillows and padding)

(5) Those areas of skin which come directly in contact with the support system are always at risk, irrespective of the method used. Great care must be taken to avoid blistering, particularly where supports are sited directly over bony prominences, such as the anterior superior iliac spines. The skin over the knees and feet must also be suitably protected. In female patients soft foam or pillows should be used to support the chest and the breasts should be displaced laterally (Smith, Gramling and Volpitto, 1961).

(6) The femoral artery, nerve and vein situated beneath the inguinal ligament should not be subjected to any compression. Some of the now out-dated support systems for the prone position which used to be inserted under the anterior superior iliac spines could become displaced medially. One or even both neuro-vascular bundles would then become trapped, with dire results.

(7) Proper support must be provided for the lower limbs. Usually a soft pad is placed under the knees and the lower legs are raised on one or two pillows. This prevents the toes from abutting on the surface of the table. The lateral cutaneous nerve of the thigh is at risk of compression damage in its subcutaneous course, as is the external popliteal nerve when it winds around the outer aspect of the neck of the fibula.

(8) In addition to the possibility of venous occlusion occurring in the groin, other such anatomical sites equally vulnerable are (*Figure 4.7*):
(a) the great veins of the neck. The chest supporting apparatus must not be allowed to override the clavicles;
(b) the liver sinusoids. It is important that the epigastrium should be completely free from the costal margin and xiphisternum downwards;
(c) the inferior vena cava should not become compressed in any way.

Preliminary anaesthetic preparations

'General anaesthesia is induced with the patient in the supine position and intubation with an armoured endotracheal tube is regarded as mandatory.' Few would argue with this dogmatic statement. In an article entitled 'Neurolept-analgesia for *awake pronation* of surgical

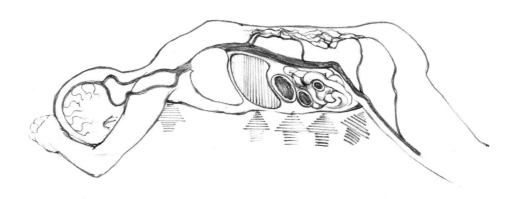

Figure 4.7 Sites where external pressure causing venous occlusion may result in engorgement of the epidural venous plexus

patients' (Lee, Barnes and Nagel, 1977) it is postulated that the risks are minimized by *awake* intubation and active cooperation by the patient in achieving the final prone position. Experience with 11 consecutive patients is described. Only two had any recollection of the incident and there were no major complaints. It is unlikely that many will adopt this technique, but it serves as a useful reminder that others have considered the risks sufficiently serious to warrant the trial of an alternative approach.

(1) In all cases a carefully secured venous access cannula should be introduced. Any fall of blood pressure following positioning the patient can be corrected rapidly then by the administration of intravenous fluids. Similarly, more sophisticated central venous or intra-arterial monitoring cannulae should be inserted whilst the patient is still supine. The addition of 'extension sets' to intravenous fluid infusion lines is often an advantage in these cases.

(2) Totally secure fixation of the endo-tracheal tube is vital to prevent accidental extubation whilst turning the patient. If adhesive strapping is used for this purpose it can become dangerously loosened by saliva draining from the mouth during the course of the operation. A mouth pack can prevent this but extra care must be taken to ensure that it is not overlooked at the end of surgery. One end should be left protruding from the mouth and the forehead should be labelled.

(3) With spontaneous respiration, impairment of ventilatory function is certain to occur in all but the shortest of surgical procedures. Most patients therefore probably require intermittent positive pressure ventilation (IPPV). If patients are to breathe spontaneously, topical analgesia to the larynx and trachea will help to prevent straining and coughing caused by inevitable movement of the endotracheal tube during the turning procedure.

(4) After induction of anaesthesia the eyes must be protected. Commercially available adhesive plasters specially shaped to cover the orbit are ideal. They must be well attached to the skin at the entire periphery in order to prevent the ingress of skin preparation fluids, aerosol plastic dressings, saliva or vomitus.

(5) Monitoring apparatus, such as ECG leads, is probably best temporarily disconnected whilst the patient is positioned, or may be placed on the back after turning.

Method of support for prone patients

There is no problem in arranging suitably placed pillows or foam pads beneath the chest and pelvis for short operations on superficial structures. This will be discussed under the heading of 'The straightforward prone position' below. The more complex procedures carried out on the posterior cranial fossae or vertebral column demand a much more sophisticated approach. Several methods have been described in the literature and, like many developments in medicine and surgery, some very similar ones have evolved more or less simultaneously in different centres. The prime objective with all of them is to eliminate completely any possibility of mechanical pressure on the large blood vessels of the groins and the abdomen, the liver sinusoids of the epigastrium and the jugular veins in the neck. This is usually achieved by ensuring that the support mechanism which is used to raise the patient above the level of the operating table exerts pressure only on bony eminences. There is, however, one notable recent development not employing this principle, and that is the use of the evacuatable mattress. In this case, supporting pressure is spread evenly under most of the anterior surface of the body.

A second and often important requirement from the surgical standpoint is good access to the interior of the intervertebral joint spaces. If the position of the patient allows any accentuation of the normal anterior lumbar lordosis, it follows that the posterior approach to the disc space will be narrowed and the surgeon may have difficulty in introducing instruments into it. Smith, Gramling and Volpitto (1961), in their description of the now obsolete 'Georgia prone position', illustrate well how rotation of the pelvis backwards and downwards, around the axis of the anterior superior iliac spine, can flatten the lumbar curve and open the posterior approach into the intervertebral disc spaces (*Figure 4.8*).

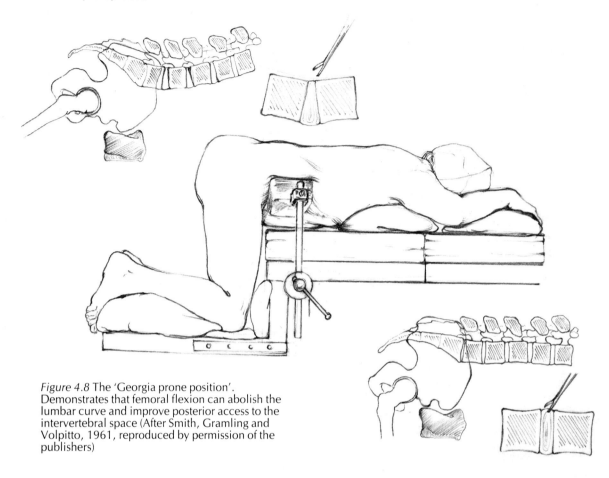

Figure 4.8 The 'Georgia prone position'.
Demonstrates that femoral flexion can abolish the
lumbar curve and improve posterior access to the
intervertebral space (After Smith, Gramling and
Volpitto, 1961, reproduced by permission of the
publishers)

The straightforward prone position

The straightforward prone position consists of
the patient having pillows or some other soft
support under the chest, pelvis and legs. It is
used only for minor surgical procedures.
Following induction of anaesthesia, the next
step is to ensure that the pillows are available
and that the team is assembled. The anaesthetist's responsibilities are to support the head and
neck, ensure continuity of the airway and to
coordinate the team. The latter must include
two strong men and at least two other persons.
The anaesthetist must ensure, by repetition if
necessary, that the assistants are absolutely
clear on the sequential steps of the procedure.
Any misunderstandings cannot be tolerated
since, apart from damage to the patient, injury
to the assistants may be incurred. Back injuries
ranging from muscle strain to prolapsed intervertebral discs are not uncommon complaints
amongst theatre technicians and nurses.

Turning into the straightforward prone position can be done in several different ways. The
authors have selected the following two-stage
method for description because they consider it
more controlled, and therefore a safer procedure.

Position of assistants (*Figure 4.9*)

(1) The anaesthetist is positioned at the head of the table supporting the patient's head and neck.

(2) The first assistant is positioned to support and turn the patient's chest.

(3) The second assistant is positioned to support and turn the pelvis and legs.

(4) The third assistant is positioned on the opposite side of the patient to place chest and pelvic supports as the patient is turned onto them.

(5) The fourth assistant looks after the legs.

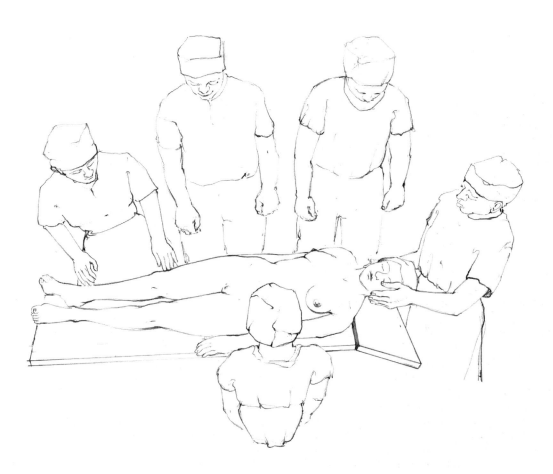

Figure 4.9 Team positions for the first stage of turning

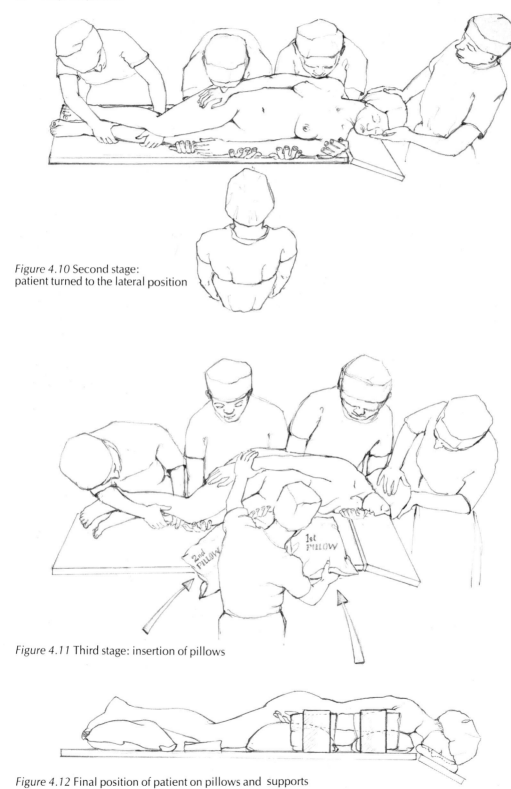

Figure 4.10 Second stage:
patient turned to the lateral position

Figure 4.11 Third stage: insertion of pillows

Figure 4.12 Final position of patient on pillows and supports

Steps in turning the patient

(1) The brakes on the operating table are secured and the head support lowered. The anaesthetist holds the head (*Figure 4.9*).

(2) The patient is lifted, rotated towards the third assistant and placed in the lateral position on the side of the table adjacent to the two main assistants. At this stage, the two main assistants do not remove their supporting arms from below the patient. The patient's lower arm is straight underneath (*Figure 4.10*).

(3) The anaesthetist lowers the table head-rest more to allow further rotation of the head without extension of the neck.

(4) The third assistant then places the chest and pelvic pillows or rubber supports on the table adjacent to the laterally positioned patient (*Figure 4.11*).

(5) Next, the patient is lifted and turned to the prone position to lie on the pillows. These are inserted in the same manoeuvre. The lower arm is taken through at the same time (*Figure 4.12*).

Final adjustments to position (*Figure 4.13*)

(1) The patient's head is supported with a soft pad or small pillow under the forehead, or possibly under the cheek with minimal rotation of the neck.

(2) The arms are supported above the head with a padded double arm-board inserted below the mattress; elbows resting on the arm-board and the forearms held by padded, right-angled arm retainers.

(3) A pillow or rubber support is placed under the knees and pillows placed under the ankles. The end-most part of the table is locked in the vertical position if head-up tilt is required.

(4) The anterior abdominal wall and particularly the epigastrium must be completely free from any pressure and should not touch the mattress even at the maximum respiratory excursion.

The diathermy plate is now applied and all monitoring and venous access lines checked. A final check is made for pressure points and metal contact. Wherever possible the final position of anaesthetic machines, monitors and infusions should be at the head-end of the table. Before the surgical drapes are applied all anaesthetic tubing connections must be tightened at each junction, equal and adequate respiratory excursion must be verified.

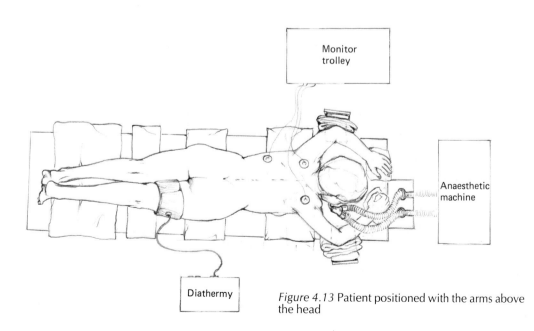

Monitor trolley

Anaesthetic machine

Diathermy

Figure 4.13 Patient positioned with the arms above the head

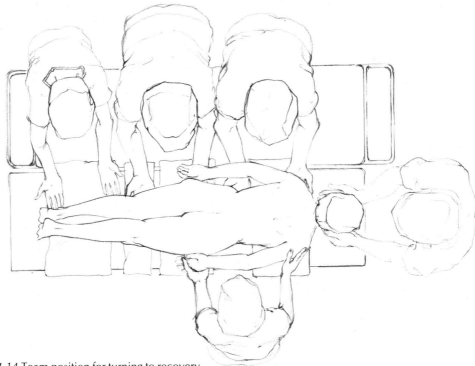

Figure 4.14 Team position for turning to recovery position and transfer to trolley

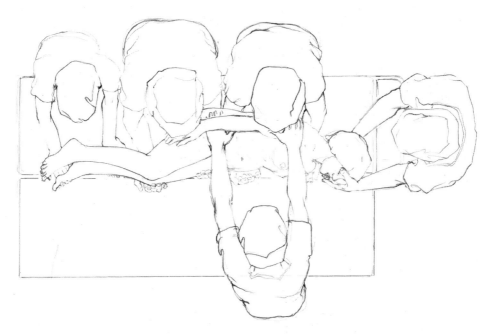

Figure 4.15 Transfer: patient retained in the lateral position for recovery

Return to the recovery position

Anaesthesia should be maintained until the patient has been turned back to the supine position. Extubation should never be done whilst the patient remains prone.

The safest and simplest procedure is to roll the patient through 90 degrees to the full lateral position and immediately effect transfer to an adjacent recovery trolley. This can be done as follows:

(1) Surgical drapes and diathermy plates are removed but anaesthetic monitoring lines are, wherever possible, left in place. It is preferable to turn the patient so that the arm with the intravenous infusion rotates above the body.

(2) The double arm-board is removed and the arms re-positioned so that the arm which will rotate beneath the body is placed alongside it.

(3) The recovery trolley is placed alongside the operating table and the wheel brakes applied. The height of the operating table is adjusted so that it is slightly above that of the trolley.

(4) The anaesthetist remains in charge of the patient's head and neck and three assistants along the free edge of the trolley extend their arms across it. They place their hands under the patient's chest, pelvis and legs (*Figure 4.14*).

(5) A fourth assistant from an opposite position then gently rolls the patient onto the arms of the lifting assistants. They retain the patient fully lateral and effect a transfer to the trolley (*Figure 4.15*).

(6) Particular care must be taken to ensure that the lower arm has been safely pulled through, and a pillow is placed under the patient's head.

Any suggestion that the prone patient be directly transferred to a ward bed, in the opinion of the authors, should be strongly resisted. Ward beds cannot always be adjusted adequately for height and their width ensures that even tall assistants have difficulty in handling the patient without imposing unwarranted strain on their own back muscles.

More complex support systems

The more complex methods of supporting prone patients currently in use fall broadly into two groups:

Group 1 Those in which the pelvis is supported or 'propped' below the anterior superior iliac spines (*Figure 4.16*).

Group II Those in which the pelvis is supported only at the ischial tuberosities (*Figure 4.17*).

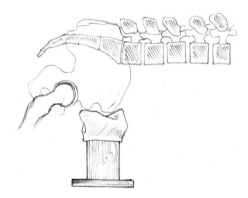

Figure 4.16 Group I methods. Support beneath the anterior superior iliac spines

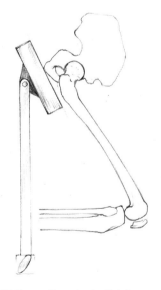

Figure 4.17 Group II methods. Pelvis supported at the ischial tuberosities

Group I methods of support

From the literature reviewed to the present, it appears that the basis of these methods stems from the work of Taylor, Gleadhill and Bilsand (1956) (*Figure 4.18*) and Pearce (1957) (*Figure 4.19*). Both these articles clearly show separate supports for each anterior superior iliac spine. They are individually adjustable on a transversely placed bar. Those described by Pearce have the advantage that they are curved at their outer margin to prevent the patient slipping sideways. The chest is supported either with pillows or a large foam rubber pad. The frame described by Smith in 1974 with great details of measurements and construction actually shows no new principles and is only a technological update of the above work (*Figure 4.20*). The pelvic supports from the Relton frame (*see below*) can be mounted on a specially made base plate (*Figure 4.21*) and function very satisfactorily when used in a similar manner. In 1967, Relton and Hall took the concept one stage further in the design of their frame for the support of patients undergoing the Harrington Rod spinal fusion procedure (*Figure 4.22*). They had found other methods unsatisfactory (Relton and Conn, 1963) and in order to prevent hyper-extension during the course of the surgery (as well as maintaining an unobstructed inferior vena cava) they mounted four well-padded adjustable props on a frame so that each could be separately positioned in order to support the chest and anterior superior iliac spines. Other workers have found this frame satisfactory for posterior fossa and cervical spinal cord surgery in otherwise skeletally normal children (Humphreys *et al.,* 1975). The Wilson frame (*Figure 4.23*) also supports both the iliac crests and the chest. It appears to be a modern version of Moore's original concept (Moore and Edmunds, 1950) but clearly does not have the versatility of Relton and Hall's design. It is really only suitable for adults having uncomplicated lumbar and lower thoracic spinal procedures. Nevertheless, there are two principal advantages. The abdomen and lower thorax are free of any pressure, which is very useful in the obese patient, and good surgical access to the intervertebral disc space is achieved by the slightly flexed posture produced. It is adjustable for both width and height, but care is needed to ensure that the operation site is at the correct level since the frame tends to 'break' asymmetrically. Precautions should be taken to ensure that it cannot slide along the surface of the table if the latter needs to be tipped. A sheepskin rug should be used to cover the surface and adjacent metal parts both to prevent pressure blisters over the iliac crests and inadvertent diathermy burns.

Figure 4.18 'Manchester' modification of Taylor's prop (1956)

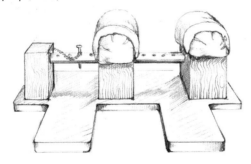

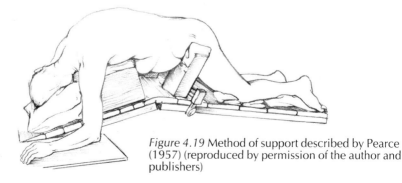

Figure 4.19 Method of support described by Pearce (1957) (reproduced by permission of the author and publishers)

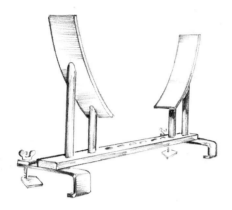

Figure 4.20 Support for pelvis as described by Smith (1974) (reproduced by permission of the author and publishers)

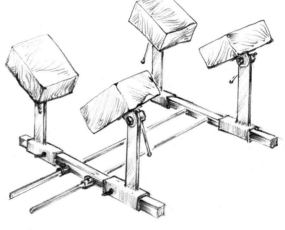

Figure 4.22 The full Relton and Hall frame designed for spinal fusion surgery using the Harrington rod (reproduced by permission of the authors and publishers)

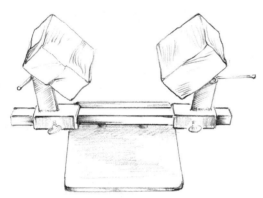

Figure 4.21 Props from the 'Relton and Hall' frame with a special base-place can be used for pelvic support in surgery on the lumbar spine

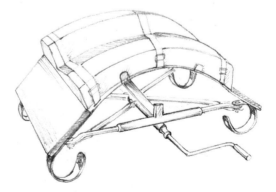

Figure 4.23 The Wilson frame

Positioning the patient

It is not necessary to deal with each of the above methods separately. The principles for all are as follows:

(1) The patient should be turned fully prone as described in the section on straightforward prone position, inserting a pillow under the chest, but omitting the pelvic support.

(2) There must be an adequate number of assistants positioned:
(a) one for each side of the patient's pelvis;
(b) at least one for the chest, depending on the weight of the patient;
(c) anaesthetist supporting the head and neck.

The patient is lifted vertically off the table, the frame inserted in the correct position and the patient gently lowered onto it. A second chest pillow or foam support may be necessary where the frame supports only the pelvis. *In all cases the neck must not be hyper-extended or over-flexed at any stage of the manoeuvre.* The face, arms and legs are supported by methods previously described: the circulation (arterial and venous) in the lower limbs is checked, external pneumatic compression apparatus should be fitted to the legs. The table should be broken, lowering the legs sufficiently (about 30 degrees) to straighten the lumbar spinal curve (*Figure 4.24*). A pendulous abdomen or male genitalia should not be allowed to remain in contact with any part of the metal support. Finally, the degree of Trendelenburg tilt is altered to ensure that the operative site is marginally above heart level.

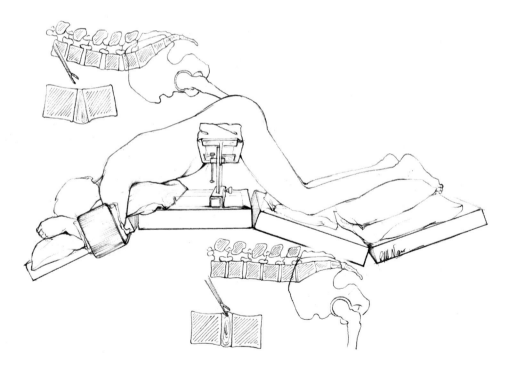

Figure 4.24 Patient positioned by Group I support method for lumbar spine surgery: see text for details

Group II methods

Here the pelvis is supported only at the ischial tuberosities. This is a development from the kneeling position described by Ecker (1949) (*Figure 4.25*) and the very similar Mohammedan prayer position (Lipton, 1950) (*Figure 4.26*), neither of which have any direct support for the pelvis. Although the latter positions have mostly been abandoned because of the excessive congestion of the lower limbs produced, which had, on occasion, resulted in renal failure from the release of myoglobin from anoxic and ischaemic muscle (Keim and Weinstein, 1970) they were, at the time of introduction, a significant advance. Prior to this, it was not unusual for patients undergoing lumbar disc surgery to be positioned with the abdomen across a metal bar in order to 'undo the anterior lumbar curve'! (Hunter, 1950).

The major advance in this position was made when it was realized that by tipping the table steeply and supporting the buttocks by a seat or sling most of the weight could be distributed in the 'sitting' mode (Tarlov, 1967; Hastings, 1969; Laurin *et al.*, 1969; Dinmore, 1977). It is important that the seat is positioned correctly under the ischial tuberosities and not the

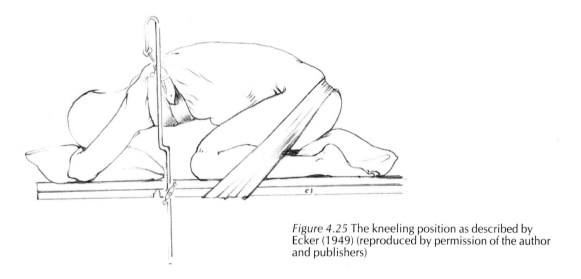

Figure 4.25 The kneeling position as described by Ecker (1949) (reproduced by permission of the author and publishers)

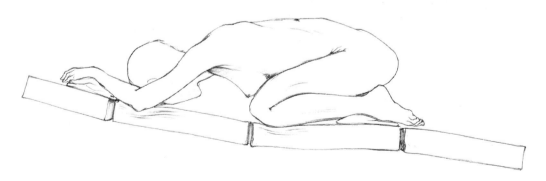

Figure 4.26 The Mohammedan Prayer position described by Lipton (1950)

femoral shafts. Some weight is obviously taken by the knees, but this is generally not sufficient to cause pressure sores or blistering. The thorax is supported by pillows, specially shaped rubber pads or a firm foam rubber roll. Again, it must be stressed that encroachment on the epigastrium or neck must not occur. These seats can be made readily in any hospital engineering workshop from the measurements illustrated (*Figure 4.27*). Wayne (1984) has reported successful experience over 15 years with this method of support.

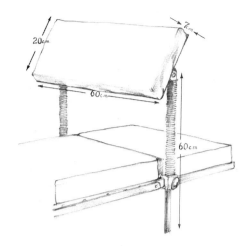

Figure 4.27 Support for ischial tuberosities in Group II methods

Positioning the patient

This position is particularly useful for lumbosacral and lower thoracic vertebral surgery. A particular advantage is its suitability for heavy patients who are difficult to position by other methods.

Positioning steps
(1) The anaesthetized patient is turned into the fully prone position as previously described.

(2) The seat is then fixed on the table with the supports at the level of the patient's knees (*Figure 4.28*).

(3) A minimum of three assistants is then required for the next phase (*Figure 4.29*) (the anaesthetist remaining in charge of the head, neck and anaesthetic hoses).
(a) Assistant 1 has responsibility for placing the chest pillows and for tipping the table steeply foot-down when ordered to do so.
(b) Assistant 2 will support the patient's chest.
(c) Assistants 3 and 4 (one on each side) will lift the patient's pelvis.

When all the assistants have been clearly instructed on their functions the anaesthetist will coordinate the patient's positioning as follows:

(1) The pelvis and chest are lifted, the knees brought below the pelvis and the patient is sat on the seat (*Figure 4.30*).

(2) As the knees are brought up below the pelvis, assistant 1 first places the chest pillows in position and then tips the table steeply foot-down to its maximum extent. This manoeuvre will result in the patient being properly supported by the ischial tuberosities on the seat itself (*Figure 4.31*).

(3) The arms and the head are then supported above the head as previously described.

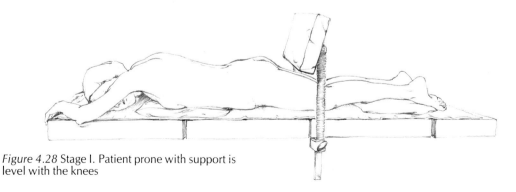

Figure 4.28 Stage I. Patient prone with support is level with the knees

Figure 4.29 Stage II. Team placings
in readiness for positioning

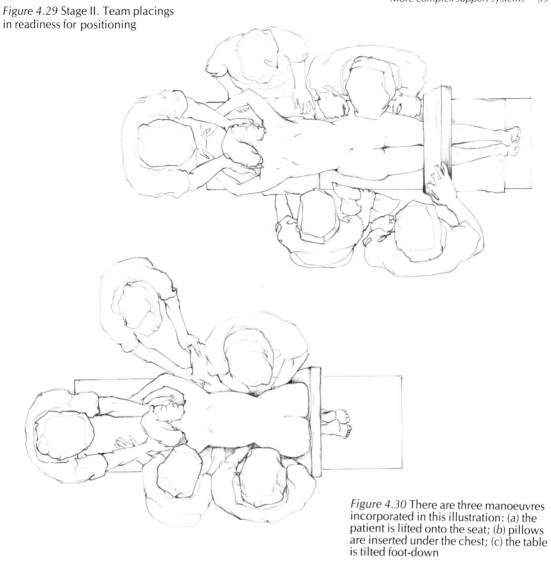

Figure 4.30 There are three manoeuvres
incorporated in this illustration: (*a*) the
patient is lifted onto the seat; (*b*) pillows
are inserted under the chest; (*c*) the table
is tilted foot-down

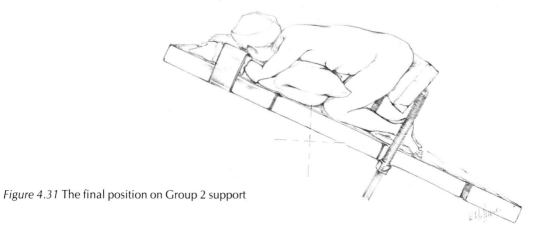

Figure 4.31 The final position on Group 2 support

Monitoring and intravenous infusions are checked and re-connected.

(4) The pneumatic leggings are placed round the lower limbs below the knees.

(5) The diathermy electrode can be conveniently sited between the patient and the seat.

(6) In heavy or very tall patients it is usually necessary to prevent the knees from slipping laterally off the side of the mattress. This can be achieved either by the use of special supports attached to the rail of the operating table, or less satisfactory, by padded 'right-angle' arm retainers inserted beneath the mattress.

(7) Final adjustments are usually necessary to the position of the chest pillows to ensure they do not encroach into the epigastrium. At first sight, this method gives a completely free anterior abdominal wall but great care should be taken to ensure that the pillows do not slip below the xiphisternum, or back pressure in the epidural veins will certainly ensue.

Position of the surgeon

The surgeon may operate from the side or from the foot-end of the table. In the latter instance some slight degree of head-up tilt may be desirable and can be achieved with some, but not all, operating tables.

Special requirements for operations on the upper thoracic and cervical vertebrae or the posterior cranial fossae

Many of these procedures are performed in the lateral or sitting position, but occasionally it is necessary to have the patient prone. In these cases it is essential that the chest is supported firmly. Group I methods may be used as may also the Relton and Hall frame (*Figure 4.32*), but Group II methods seldom allow enough 'head-up tilt' to give good operating conditions. The 'Concorde position' (*Figure 4.33*) has been described recently for intracranial surgery in the prone position (Kobayshi *et al.*, 1983). The head is both flexed and higher than heart level. The authors cannot comment on its efficacy.

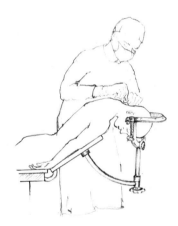

Figure 4.33 The 'Concorde position' as described by Kobayshi *et al.* (1983) (reproduced by permission of the authors and publishers)

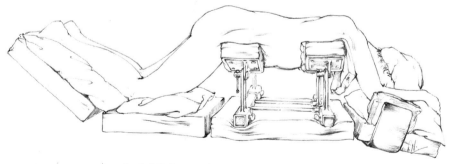

Figure 4.32 Patient supported on the full Relton and Hall frame. The upper supportes are as close as possible to the midline. The lower supports are wider apart and are each centred on the anterior superior iliac spines

References

Batson, O. V. (1940) The function of the vertebral veins and their role in the spread of metastasis. *Annals of Surgery,* **112**, 139–149

Britt, B. A. and Gordon, R. A. (1964) Peripheral nerve injuries associated with anaesthesia. *Canadian Anaesthetists Society Journal,* **11**, 514–536

Dinmore, P. (1977) A new operating position for posterior spinal surgery. *Anaesthesia, 32,* 377–380

Ecker, A. (1949) Kneeling position for operations on the lumbar spine. Especially for protruded intervertebral disc. *Surgery,* **25**, 112

Hastings, D. E. (1969) A simple frame for operations on the lumbar spine. *Canadian Journal of Surgery,* **12**, 251–253

Humphreys, R. P., Creigton, R. E., Hendrick, E. B. and Hoffman, H. J. (1975) Advantages of the prone position for neurosurgical procedures on the upper cervical spine and posterior cranial fossa in children. *Childs Brain,* **1**, 325–336

Hunter, A. R. (1950) Anaesthesia for operations in the vertebral canal. *Anesthesiology,* **12**, 367–373

Keim, H. A. and Weinstein, J. D. (1970) Acute renal failure. A complication of spine fusion in the Tuck position. *Journal of Bone and Joint Surgery,* **52Aii**, 1248–1250

Kobayshi, S., Sugita, K., Tanaka, Y. and Kyoshima, K. (1983) Infratentorial approach to the pineal region in the prone position: Concorde position. *Journal of Neurosurgery,* **58**, 141–143

Laurin, C. A., Migneault, G., Brunet, J. L. and Roy, P. (1969) Knee-chest support for lumbosacral operations. *Canadian Journal of Surgery,* **12**, 225–250

Lee, C., Barnes, A. and Nagel, E. L. (1977) Neuroleptanalgesia for awake pronation of surgical patients. *Anesthesia and Analgesia,* **56**, 276–278

Lipton, S. (1950) Anaesthesia in the surgery of retropulsed vertebral discs. *Anaesthesia,* **5**, 208–212

Mixter, J. M. and Barr, J. S. (1934) Rupture of the intervertebral disc with involvement of the spinal canal. *New England Journal of Medicine,* **211**, 210–214

Moore, D. C. and Edmunds, L. H. (1950) Prone position frame. *Surgery,* **27**, 276–279

Norgore, M. (1945) Clinical anatomy of the vertebral veins. *Surgery,* **17**, 606–615

Pearce, D. J. (1957) The role of posture in laminectomy. *Proceedings of the Royal Society of Medicine,* **50**, 109–112

Relton, J. E. S. and Conn, A. W. (1963) Anaesthesia for the surgical correction of scoliosis by the Harrington method in children. *Canadian Anaesthetists Society Journal,* **10**, 603–615

Relton, J. E. S. and Hall, J. E. (1967) An operation frame for spinal fusion. A new apparatus designed to reduce haemorrhage during operation. *Journal of Bone and Joint Surgery,* **49B**, 327–332

Smith, R. H. (1974) One solution to the problem of the prone position for surgical procedures. *Anesthesia and Analgesia,* **53**, 221–224

Smith, R. H., Gramling, Z. W. and Volpitto, P. P. (1961) Problems related to the prone position for surgical operations. *Anesthesiology,* **22**, 189–193

Tarlov, I. M. (1967) The knee–chest position for lower spinal operations. *Journal of Bone and Joint Surgery,* **49A**, 1193–1194

Taylor, A. R., Gleadhill, C. A. and Bilsand, W. L. (1956) Posture and anaesthesia for spinal operations with special reference to intervertebral disc surgery. *British Journal of Anaesthesia,* **28**, 213–219

Wayne, S. J. (1984) A modification of the tuck position for lumbar spine surgery. A 15-year follow-up study. *Clinical Orthopaedics,* **184**, 212–216

Chapter five

The sitting position

T. V. Campkin

This chapter is concerned with the use of the sitting position during major surgery; such surgery almost invariably involves a neurosurgical exploration either of an occipital lobe, the most posterior part of a cerebral hemisphere or of the posterior cranial (infratentorial) fossa. The latter compartment contains the lower part of the brain stem (pons and medulla oblongata), the cerebellum and the lower cranial nerves. Within the brain stem are sited the vital centres that control respiration and cardiovascular function as well as lower cranial nerve nuclei.

Apart from intracranial procedures, the sitting position is also often preferred for operations on the cervical spine. Although, in the United Kingdom, patients who require outpatient dental operations of short duration (usually exodontia) are sometimes anaesthetized sitting up, such procedures will not be considered here.

Less risk is incurred by placing the patient prone or semi-prone, a position which allows access to the posterior fossa and cervical spine; nevertheless, in many centres, the sitting position is still widely used. In the past, there were good reasons for this preference because the standard of general anaesthesia was often less than satisfactory; in the sitting position relatively good operating conditions were provided for the surgeon. Respiration was not impeded, the venous pressure was low and cerebral congestion tended to be less than when the patient was lying down. However, even today, despite the use of controlled ventilation and improved neuro-anaesthesia techniques, the sitting position has retained its popularity. In a recent survey in just over half the institutions

in the United Kingdom, it was still routinely used for posterior fossa explorations (Campkin, 1981), while among North American centres it would appear that the proportion favouring the sitting position is higher. Apart from reduced operative haemorrhage, both arterial and venous, and a relatively uncongested brain, other advantages claimed for the surgeon are that, with the patient upright and the head well flexed, good access and visualization from directly behind is possible rather than above and from one side which is the case if the patient is lying prone. From the anaesthetist's point of view, it allows easy access to the tracheal tube and also for intravenous fluid administration. Moreover, if general anaesthesia with spontaneous respiration is maintained, and there are occasional circumstances when this may be desirable, breathing will be unimpeded.

Anatomical hazards and other complications

Nerve lesions

Faulty positioning or prolonged surgery can lead to peripheral nerve lesions. The arms must be well supported and any traction on the neck avoided: brachial plexus damage has been reported (Saady, 1981). Ulnar nerve compression can occur at the elbow if the ulnar groove is in contact with the edge of the operating table or compressed by an arm support. Bilateral paresis of the common peroneal nerves which resulted in foot drop has also followed a prolonged craniotomy (Keykah and Rosenberg, 1979). The lateral aspect of the knees must not be in contact with the head-holding frame and the feet should be maintained in a median position of dorsiflexion. The sciatic nerve may be stretched if the thighs are flexed to a right angle while the knees remain fully extended (Bedford, 1983). Finally, the combination of flexion and rotation of the cervical spine and prolonged focal pressure can lead to damage to the spinal cord (Hitselberger and House, 1980). These authors cite five cases of quadriplegia that followed acoustic neuroma surgery; in one patient autopsy revealed infarction of the mid-cervical cord, possibly related to a previously unrecognized spondylitic bar at the level of the infarction.

Orthopaedic and cutaneous lesions

Two cases of haemarthrosis and dislocation of the elbow occurred in a large series of patients who were anaesthetized in the sitting position (Standefer, Bay and Trusso, 1984). In the same series four patients developed pressure excoriation of the skin in the lumbosacral region following prolonged surgery; a fifth sustained pressure damage to the skin of the forehead, from a cerebellar head-rest. Such complications, although unusual, emphasize the importance of careful positioning of the limbs and the need for adequate protective padding during long operations.

Airway complications

The possibility of traction on the tracheal tube by the anaesthetic hose, and of migration of the tip of the tube downwards when the head is flexed, is discussed later. Although it is customary to insert an oropharyngeal airway after intubation, oedema and swelling of the tongue have followed the use of one during a long procedure in the sitting position (McAllister, 1974; Ellis, Bryan-Brown and Hyderally, 1975). It has also been reported in cases where no oropharyngeal mouthpack or airway was used (Tattersall, 1984; Munshi, Dhamee and Gandhi, 1984). It is probably associated with extremes of neck flexion.

Fall in body temperature

The sitting position allows the patient to be exposed to draughts and this can be a particular problem in children in whom the body temperature may fall rapidly. Apart from warming intravenous infusion fluid to body temperature, the child should be well wrapped with blankets and a metallized plastic sheet (space blanket).

Cardiovascular complications

Postural hypotension may occur when the patient is sitting up and will be worsened by operative haemorrhage and by intermittent positive pressure ventilation, which tends to reduce venous return and hence cardiac output. It is recommended that patients considered liable to develop hypotension should not be sat up but if the sitting position is essential the use of leg bandages and keeping the knees flexed at heart level will help to maintain venous return.

Intra-operative cranial nerve or brain stem manipulation may produce sudden changes in blood pressure (either hypotension or hypertension) and heart rate or the appearance of cardiac dysrhythmias. Surgical retractor pressure or the use of the electrocautery in the vicinity of the brain stem usually cause a bradycardia and fall in blood pressure which will be accentuated in the sitting position. The wide variety of electrocardiographic (ECG) changes that can occur include conduction abnormalities and supraventricular or ventricular ectopic beats. Although such changes all suggest serious interference with brain stem function, they are usually transient and provided that the surgeon is informed, and that he ceases manipulation, the heart rate and blood pressure usually quickly return to normal.

Venous air embolism (VAE)

VAE has been recognized as a cause of sudden death during surgery in the head-up or sitting position for more than 150 years but until comparatively recently it was regarded as a rare, although often lethal, complication. However, with the development of sensitive methods to detect the presence of small volumes of air in the circulation it has become clear that this is a frequent occurrence; using an ultrasonic probe (Maroon, Edmonds-Seal and Campbell, 1969) or end-tidal CO_2 monitoring (Brechner and Bethune, 1971) the reported incidence is 20–40 per cent.

For air to gain entry to the circulation, there must be an open and uncollapsed vein in which there is a negative venous pressure and this situation may exist during operation in the sitting position. The most usual portals of entry are veins which traverse bone (diploic and emissary) or those in which the outer, adventitious coat is fused to the periosteum or ligaments of cervical vertebrae. Thus, this complication usually, but not always, occurs during bone removal at an early stage of the operation.

Adequate monitoring to detect VAE at an early stage and the insertion of a right atrial catheter, is mandatory and is discussed below. Immediately the diagnosis is made, the surgeon should be informed and the wound flooded with saline or a large moist pack inserted in order to prevent the entry of further air. All anaesthetic agents are discontinued, 100 per cent oxygen administered and air is aspirated as rapidly as possible from the heart via the right atrial catheter.

Early detection and prompt treatment will usually avoid a serious fall in pressure, but if this occurs the period for which the patient can remain in the sitting position is strictly limited. Thus, if a systolic pressure of at least 80 mmHg has not been restored within 2.5 minutes, the patient must be placed recumbent, a manoeuvre which involves team work in order to avoid contamination of the surgical field. The surgical field is covered with sterile dressing, the head is removed from its fixing device, the chair rapidly converted back into an operating table and the patient placed in the semi-prone position.

Finally, to prevent VAE, a simple prophylactic measure comprises intermittent manual compression by the anaesthetist of the jugular veins at the root of the neck. This is carried out at the surgeon's request at intervals during the early stages of the operation and helps to identify open veins which are not bleeding.

Choice between sitting and prone or lateral positions

Before deciding whether the patient should be sitting for cranial or cervical spinal surgery it is important to discuss with the surgeon the relative advantages and disadvantages of this posture. Thus, it may be unwise to place seriously ill patients in this position, particularly if the level of consciousness is obtunded due to raised intracranial pressure (ICP), or if they have marked ataxia. Such patients may have been confined to bed for a prolonged period and in these circumstances vasomotor tone, which helps to maintain the blood pressure in the erect position, is often impaired. Hypovolaemia due to vomiting or decreased fluid intake can also lead to marked arterial hypotension. The sitting position is unsuitable, even when ICP is not raised, for those patients who are elderly, debilitated or suffering from ischaemic heart disease or severe arterial hypertension, particularly if they are also receiving medication with beta-adrenergic blocking drugs or calcium antagonists. A significant proportion of elderly patients with cervical spondylosis who require decompressive surgery fall into this group and marked hypotension can occur when they are placed in the sitting position.

Finally, although the sitting position is widely used for posterior fossa explorations in children, it is not satisfactory for those under three to four years of age. For such cases, the prone or semi-prone positions are preferable.

Important aspects of anaesthesia and monitoring

The choice of premedication and intravenous induction agents, both narcotic drugs and muscle relaxants, has relevance to the proposed position of the patient during surgery. Although these are a matter of personal preference and will not be discussed in detail, agents should be used which do not predispose to arterial hypotension. It is also worth mentioning that intramuscular atropine should be included in the premedication. The decrease in salivation is helpful because, when the patient is placed upright without an antisialogogue being used, secretions from the mouth can loosen the fixation of the tracheal tube.

The type of tracheal tube used is also of importance. This should not kink or be easily compressed, and in the past it has been routine practice to use a re-sterilizable latex tube, reinforced by a metal spiral, the so-called 'armoured latex' tube. However, during the last few years, disposable PVC tubes with high volume, low pressure cuffs, have been found to be equally satisfactory. Recently PVC tubes which incorporate a reinforcing spiral have also been introduced.

When upright, the patient's head will usually be well flexed and maintained in position, using a head-rest or skull-holding device but, even when maximally flexed, a space of at least 2.5 cm should be left between the chin and the sternum. In this position, a tracheal tube, the tip of which may have been correctly sited at induction, tends to migrate further down the trachea, and may then impact at the carina or even pass into the right main bronchus. This complication will be avoided if the tube is introduced no more than 5.0 cm into the trachea, and half this distance in children.

A moistened pharyngeal pack is often used to stabilize the tracheal tube and the insertion of an oropharyngeal airway will prevent compression of the tube by the patient's teeth. The eyes are protected by vaseline gauze covered with lint and adhesive strapping against abrasion or the accidental entry of antiseptic solutions used to clean the scalp.

Monitoring

Accurate monitoring of the cardiovascular system is essential, which implies a continuous display of blood pressure, heart rate and the ECG. For blood pressure measurement, a 1.0 mm non-tapered teflon cannula is inserted into the radial artery of the non-dominant limb. When the patient is seated, the transducer should be sited and calibrated at the level of the base of the skull, so that the inflow pressure to the cerebral arterial system is measured. Alternatively, the observed pressure reading can be corrected by deducting 2.0 mmHg for each 2.5 cm of vertical height between the transducer and the base of the skull.

Several monitoring techniques are available for the early detection of VAE. Of these, the Doppler ultrasonic probe and the continuous measurement of respired carbon dioxide (FE_{CO_2}) are the most widely used and in many centres are considered essential. Using the Doppler device, an ultrasonic beam, generated by a piezo-electric crystal, is reflected by moving red cells, and received by a second crystal. The change in frequency between the transmitted and reflected ultrasound is amplified and displayed as an audible flow signal. If even a small volume of air enters the circulation, the blood–air interface is an excellent reflector of ultrasound and there is an abrupt change in the character of the flow sounds. This may be an isolated 'chirp' or a more continuous scraping noise.

The Doppler probe, coated with acoustic gel, is positioned at the right side of the sternum: the loudest flow sounds are usually heard between the third and sixth interspace. Alternatively, the left mid-sternal border is chosen and in this position the pulmonary outflow tract is monitored. Frequently, it is necessary to reposition the probe when the patient is fully seated, since it may become displaced during the moving process. The principal disadvantage of this apparatus is that the use of the electrocautery causes total interference and most modern equipment incorporates a deactivating device which suppresses its action when the diathermy is in use. Further drawbacks are that the hirsute male chest or pendulous breasts sometimes make it extremely difficult to position the probe firmly.

An infrared analyser is used to monitor respired CO_2 and this should be displayed on a slow moving chart recorder. A sudden fall in the end-tidal concentration ($F_{ET}CO_2$) should be presumed to be due to VAE. CO_2 measurement is unaffected by the diathermy but it should be emphasized that operative haemorrhage, which causes a decrease in cardiac output and hence pulmonary blood flow, will also reduce $F_{ET}CO_2$. However, such change is usually more gradual in onset than when VAE occurs.

A central venous catheter should be placed in the right atrium and an approach from the antecubital fossa, preferably via the basilic vein, is routinely used. It is necessary to confirm, by chest radiography, and before the patient is sat up, that the catheter is correctly sited. If chest radiography is not possible, an alternative method of verifying the position of the catheter tip is to place the Doppler probe to the right of the sternal border and rapidly inject 5 ml of heparinized saline. If correctly sited, an immediate alteration of Doppler flow sounds is heard (Tinker *et al.*, 1975).

Similar monitoring is necessary for children undergoing posterior fossa procedures, although in such cases it is preferred to place the atrial catheter via the internal jugular vein. A soft Seldinger catheter can be taped down on the chest and does not interfere with the surgical access (Beasley, 1986). The possibility of an undesirable fall in body temperature has already been noted and the oesophageal temperature should be monitored.

Finally, certain more sophisticated monitoring techniques have been described. These include the insertion of a flow-directed pulmonary artery catheter which permits aspiration of air as well as indicating the volume embolized (Marshall and Bedford, 1980). A transoesophageal Doppler probe has also been used with success in dogs (Martin and Colley, 1983) while detection of VAE by transoesophageal echocardiography is claimed to be both sensitive and accurate (Cucchiara *et al.*, 1984).

Steps in positioning the patient

Adequate personnel, who are familiar with the procedure, must be available to move the anaesthetized patient from a trolley onto an operating table which can then be converted into a 'chair'. The standard operating table-top has four components, i.e. two central sections which can be angled, and removable head and foot sections. The following steps are necessary before the patient is fully sat up.

(1) The patient is placed on the operating table with the iliac crests above the central break. The head is temporarily supported on a horseshoe head-rest (*Figure 5.1*). It is particularly important in patients with cervical spondylosis that there is no undue flexion, extension or rotation of the neck. The blood pressure should be checked, and it is a wise precaution to have a vasoconstrictor drug (e.g. methoxamine or metaraminol) available in the event of undue hypotension occurring when the patient is sat up.

(2) The central section of the operating table is now flexed until it becomes almost a right angle (*Figure 5.2*). This should be done slowly, the sitting position being gradually reached over a period of 5 minutes. The blood pressure is carefully monitored throughout.

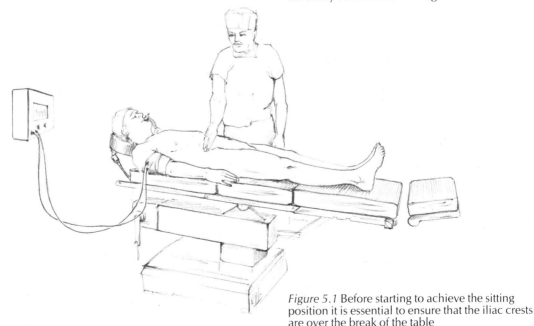

Figure 5.1 Before starting to achieve the sitting position it is essential to ensure that the iliac crests are over the break of the table

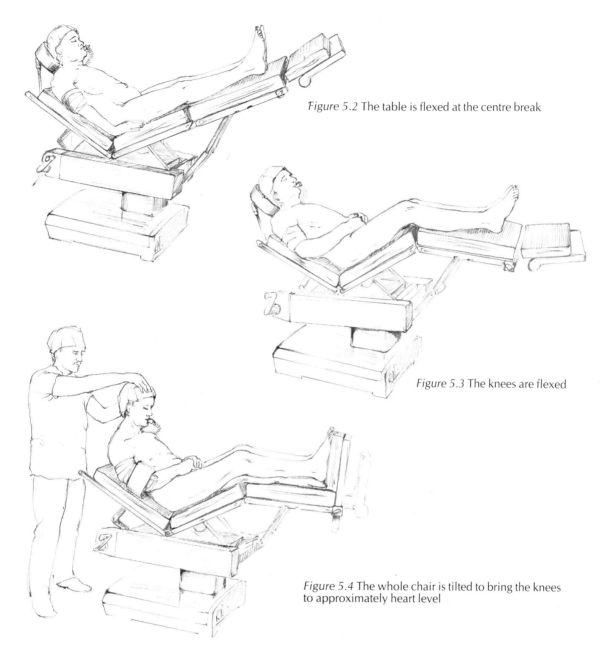

Figure 5.2 The table is flexed at the centre break

Figure 5.3 The knees are flexed

Figure 5.4 The whole chair is tilted to bring the knees to approximately heart level

(3) When sitting, the patient's buttocks must be well positioned into the angle formed by the central section, so that there is no tendency to slide forward (*Figure 5.3*). The thighs are flexed at right angles to the trunk.

(4) The foot-end of the operating table is broken so that the patient's knees are slightly flexed and rest on a pillow. The legs are also supported by a pillow with the feet in a median position of dorsiflexion.

(5) The arms are supported by padded arm-rests and the elbows flexed so that the forearms rest across the patient's abdomen.

(6) Finally, the whole chair is tilted backwards to bring the knees level, or almost level, with the patient's heart (*Figure 5.4*).

Figure 5.5 Patient in position using three-pin clamp

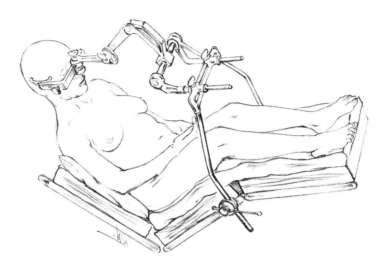

Positioning the head

In the past, a horseshoe-shaped cerebellar head-rest has been popular. A more satisfactory and widely used head-holder consists of a C-shaped device that incorporates sterilizable metal pins, which pierce the outer table of the skull; one of the most popular is the Mayfield clamp (*Figure 5.5*). Using this pin-type head holder there is no risk of orbital or soft tissue pressure and it is easier to rotate the head for lateral explorations. For most posterior fossa procedures, the patient's head should be well flexed, although, as already noted, a space should be left between the chin and the sternum. Less flexion is required for operations on the cervical spine, and indeed undue flexion in such cases may be dangerous (*see below*).

Once the head is positioned, the anaesthetic hose should be lightly fixed to the head-rest frame, in order to avoid traction on the tracheal tube. Care should also be taken that no part of the metal frame is in contact with the patient's skin.

Return to the supine position

At the completion of surgery in the sitting position, it is important to maintain controlled ventilation and an adequate depth of anaesthesia until the patient has been returned to the supine position. In particular, an episode of coughing or straining on the tracheal tube while the head is still fixed and relatively inaccessible to the anaesthetist must be avoided, since this will lead to cerebral congestion and possibly a dangerous rise in ICP.

The head, freed from its fixing device (which is removed), is supported by the surgeon while dressings are applied. The head-end of the operating table is now replaced and the 'chair' converted back to the standard horizontal operating table. A pillow is placed beneath the patient's head. Muscle relaxation is now reversed, anaesthesia lightened and the tracheal tube removed once spontaneous respiration is deemed adequate.

The 'side-saddle' position

With the patient positioned as described above, it is difficult to return the patient rapidly to the supine position if this should become necessary. A variation of the conventional sitting position has, therefore, been recommended (Garcia-Bengochea, Munson and Freeman, 1976) (*Figure 5.6*). This involves extensive adaptation of an operating table so that the patient sits in a lateral or 'side-saddle' position. In the event of serious hypotension or VAE, the lateral horizontal position can be quickly obtained without the need to remove the patient's head from its fixing device or disturbance and possible contamination of the operating site (*Figure 5.7*).

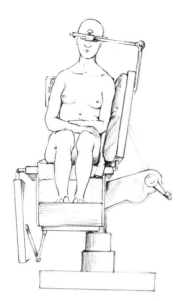

Figure 5.6 'Side saddle' position upright (After Garcia-Bengochea *et al.*, 1976, by permission of the authors and publishers)

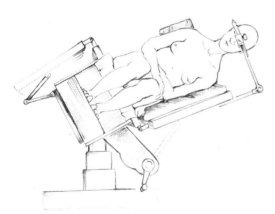

Figure 5.7 'Side saddle' position tipped to horizontal (After Garcia-Bengochea *et al.*, 1976, by permission of the authors and publishers)

References

Beasley, J. (1986) Anaesthesia for neurosurgery in children. In *Neurosurgical Anaesthesia and Intensive Care*, 2nd edn, pp. 254–267. Edited by T. V. Campkin and J. M. Turner. Butterworths, London

Bedford, R. F. (1983) Posterior fossa procedures. In *Handbook of Neuroanaesthesia. Clinical and Physiologic Essentials*, pp. 247–259. Edited by P. Newfield and J. E. Cottrell. Little, Brown, Boston

Brechner, V. L. and Bethune, R. W. N. (1971) Recent advances in monitoring pulmonary air embolism. *Anesthesia and Analgesia Current Researches*, **50**, 225–261

Campkin, T. V. (1981) Posture and ventilation during posterior fossa and cervical operations. *British Journal of Anaesthesia*, **53**, 881–884

Cucchiara, R. F., Nugent, M., Seward, J. B. and Messick, J. M. (1984) Air embolism in upright neurosurgical patients: Detection and localization by two-dimensional trans-oesophageal echocardiography. *Anesthesiology*, **60**, 353–355

Ellis, S. C., Bryan-Brown, C. W. and Hyderally, M. (1975) Massive swelling of the head and neck. *Anesthesiology*, **42**, 102–103

Garcia-Bengochea, F., Munson, E. S. and Freeman, J. V. (1976) The lateral sitting position for neurosurgery. *Anesthesia and Analgesia Current Researches*, **55**, 326–330

Hitselberger, W. E. and House, W. S. A. (1980) Warning regarding the sitting position for acoustic tumour surgery. *Archives of Otolaryngology*, **106**, 69

Keykah, M. M. and Rosenberg, H. (1974) Bilateral footdrop after craniotomy in the sitting position. *Anesthesiology*, **51**, 163–164

McAllister, R. G. (1974) Macroglossia – a positional complication. *Anesthesiology*, **40**, 199–200

Maroon, J. C., Edmonds-Seal, J. and Campbell, R. L. (1969) An ultrasonic method for detecting air embolism. *Journal of Neurosurgery*, **31**, 196–201

Marshall, W. K. and Bedford, R. F. (1980) Use of a pulmonary artery catheter for detection and treatment of venous air embolism. A prospective study in man. *Anesthesiology*, **52**, 131–134

Martin, R. W. and Colley, P. S. (1983) Evaluation of transoesophageal Doppler detection of air embolism in dogs. *Anesthesiology*, **58**, 117–123

Munshi, C. A., Dhamee, M. S. and Gandhi, S. K. (1984) Postoperative unilateral facial oedema: a complication of acute flexion of the neck. *Canadian Anaesthetists Society Journal*, **31**, 197–199

Saady, A. (1981) Brachial plexus palsy after anaesthesia in the sitting position. *Anaesthesia*, **36**, 194–195

Standefer, M., Bay, J. W. and Trusso, R. (1984) The sitting position in neurosurgery: a retrospective analysis of 488 cases. *Neurosurgery*, **14**, 649–658

Tattersall, M. P. (1984) Massive swelling of the face and tongue. A complication of posterior fossa surgery in the sitting position. *Anaesthesia*, **39**, 1015–1017

Tinker, J. H., Gronert, G. A., Messick, J. M. and Michelfelder, J. D. (1975) Detection of air embolism. A test for positioning of right atrial catheter and Doppler probe. *Anesthesiology*, **43**, 104–106

Chapter six

The transfer of patients and recovery room practice

Patients are transferred to the operating theatre either in their beds or by specially designed trolley. Account may need to be taken of their general condition; modification of the usual routine is sometimes needed in those who are very sick or have major fractures. Conventionally, the majority of patients arrive at theatre in the supine position but those for Caesarean section should always be transported in the fully lateral or 'wedged' position.

Prior to the induction of anaesthesia, privacy and the maintenance of dignity are especially important. All unnecessary exposure must be avoided and every aspect of modesty should be respected. Edentulous patients in particular, are often extremely embarrassed under such conditions and anxious even to avoid being seen by their own relatives.

Once the patient arrives in the operating theatre, safe transfer is the responsibility of the anaesthetist.

Hazards encountered with transfer systems

Damage to the cervical spine

'Whiplash' injury is a well-recognized accident occurring as a result of careless transfer of the sedated or unconscious patient. It can happen whenever the unsupported head is allowed to fall backwards or sideways.

(1) This may occur when the supporting canvas stretcher has been incorrectly placed beneath the patient and its upper margin is only level with the shoulders (*Figure 6.1*). A pillow

placed beneath the patient's head can hide this so that when the patient is lifted, the pillow slips away between the poles and the head falls backwards.

(2) Uncoordinated and over-enthusiastic turning of the patient from the supine to any other position without the head being correctly held can also result in abnormal stress on the cervical vertebrae (*Figure 6.2*). It occurs not infrequently in the recovery room.

It must be stressed that, with any sedated or unconscious patient, the head and neck must be firmly supported at every stage of patient transfer or change of position.

Accidents in which the patient falls to the floor

At any stage of transfer there is the possibility that the patient may fall to the floor. No serious harm may ensue (Farman, 1978) but the potential for serious or fatal injury is obvious. The circumstances leading to this mishap are often of multiple aetiology involving at least one of the following factors:

(1) An insecure receiving trolley. Failure to apply the brakes or raise the guard rail on the far side are elementary mistakes. Absence of an assistant specifically positioned to steady the trolley would also be a contributing factor (*Figure 6.3*).

(2) Inadequate physique of the lifting attendants relative to the weight of the patient. The patients then tend to be dragged across rather

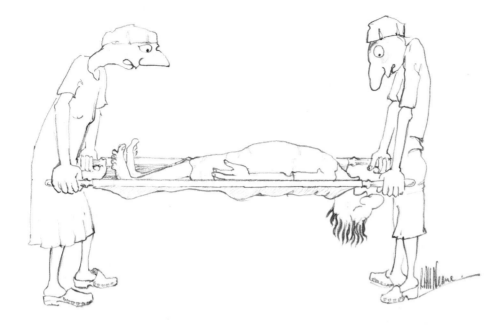

Figure 6.1 It is essential that the stretcher canvas supports the head and neck

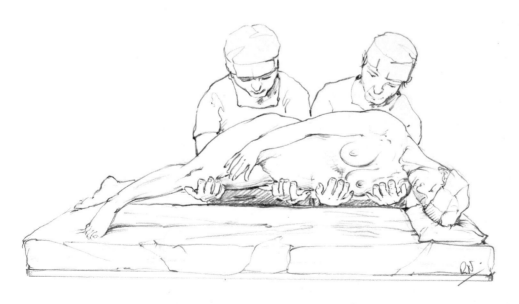

Figure 6.2 Turning the patient without supporting the head may result in damage to the cervical spine

72

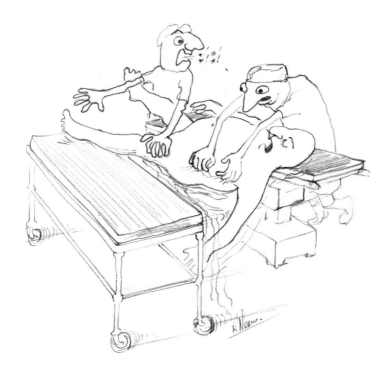

Figure 6.3 The brakes on the recovery trolley must be
applied and the trolley secured

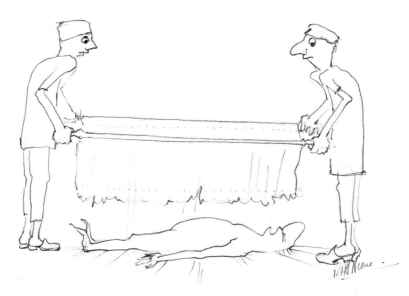

Figure 6.4 The stretcher canvas must be in good
condition

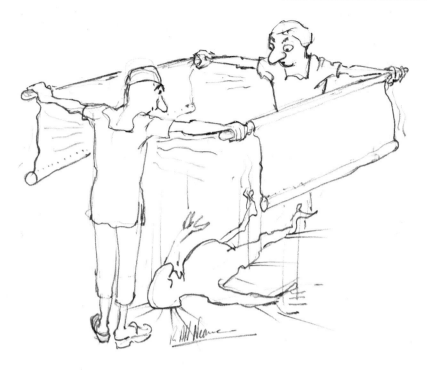

Figure 6.5 Ensure that only one canvas is placed beneath the patient

than cleanly lifted and this can push the receiving trolley away from the operating table.

(3) Faults with the stretcher canvas. There are two possibilities here:

(a) A badly worn canvas may tear longitudinally down one edge allowing the pole to become free and the patient to fall through (*Figure 6.4*).

(b) The second hazard occurs when two canvases have been placed inadvertently on top of one another beneath the patient. If one pole is then mistakenly placed in each canvas the patient may then be partially lifted and moved before falling between the two (*Figure 6.5*).

(4) Misalignment of transfer trolley tops to pedestals of operating table bases. Slight misalignment may remain unnoticed until the operating table is raised or lowered or until a surgical assistant leans against it. The patient can then be promptly precipitated towards the floor (*Figure 6.6*).

(5) Failure to raise both guard rails, particularly on narrow trolleys. Semiconscious patients recovering from anaesthesia are particularly at risk. If the patient is recovering in bed an attendant should be present constantly (and guard rails used if necessary) until the patient is conscious and reasonably orientated.

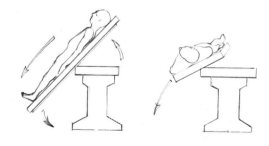

Figure 6.6 It is vital to ensure that operating table tops are correctly aligned and secured to the fixed table base

Damage to the upper limbs

(1) When stretcher poles are inserted along the canvas from the foot-end of the patient the olecranon process can be fractured or badly bruised (*Figure 6.7*). It is particularly vulnerable if the arms are folded across the chest because then it is in a direct line with the ascending pole unless deliberately raised by an assistant.

(2) The fingers should never be allowed to hang freely at the sides; digits have been crushed or amputated accidently when placing patients on some of the sophisticated transfer top operating tables.

Figure 6.7 When inserting a stretcher pole the patient's elbows must be lifted

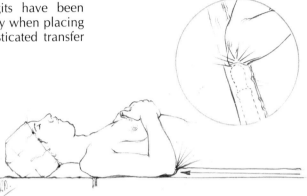

Skin damage

This may result from careless removal of a rough canvas stretcher from beneath the patient. Usually the patient is turned into the lateral position and that part of the canvas so revealed is rolled longitudinally towards the centre of the bed. The patient is then rotated onto the other side. It should then be possible to withdraw the stretcher cover gently. If care is not taken, abrasions or even skin burns can be produced (*Figure 6.8*).

Figure 6.8 The stretcher canvas must be removed gently

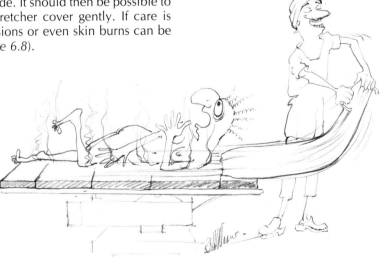

Damage from accidental traction to infusion lines, drainage tubes and catheters (*Figure* 6.9)

(1) Intermittent re-use intravenous needles of the 'butterfly' type are easily dislodged during patient transfer. Surveys of this type of device have shown that at least 15 per cent (Harvey, 1983; Sale, 1984) are no longer functional by the time the patient reaches the recovery room. Tully *et al.* (1981) showed an overall 'cut out' rate (with extravasation of injected fluids) of 40 per cent with respect to steel needles. If a subcutaneous injection of drugs is given through a misplaced needle, the consequences may be serious and have resulted in successful litigation (Green, 1981).

(2) Intravenous cannulae attached to infusion lines may be pulled out completely when the patient is moved if the infusion bag remains anchored to the drip stand or if the tubing is trapped. The patient will be left with an unsightly haematoma and the anaesthetist with the necessity of resiting the cannula.

(3) Wound and peritoneal cavity vacuum drainage containers may become detached from their tubing. Sterility is thus compromised, and a secondary infection may follow. Glass bottles used for this purpose may be broken and pose a hazard for theatre staff.

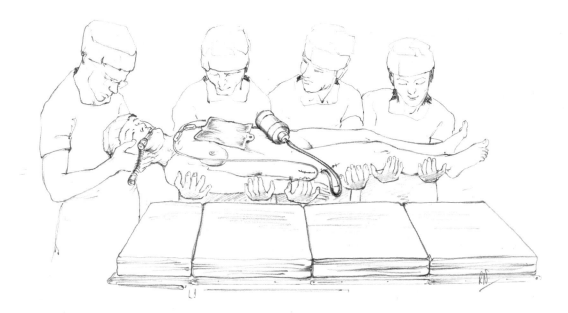

Figure 6.9 All infusion lines, catheters and drains must be free to move with the patient

(4) Correct management and care of chest drainage bottles and tubing is mandatory during patient transfer. The proximal part of the tube must be double-clamped prior to any move from the operating table (*Figure 6.10*). Any failure of the cross-clamping subjects the patient to two hazards:

(a) Air may enter the pleural cavity causing a pneumothorax should the bottle break, or the tubing become detached.
(b) Fluid from the underwater drain may be syphoned into the patient's chest if the drainage container is inadvertently raised above the level of the patient (*Figure 6.11*).

Figure 6.10 Chest drains must be double-clamped before transfer

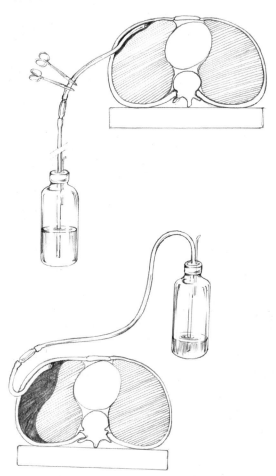

Figure 6.11 An unclamped drainage bottle must never be raised above the patient

(5) Damage to the urethra. Indwelling urinary catheters are retained in position by the use of an inflatable balloon situated in the bladder. If the drainage bag to which the catheter is attached remains anchored to the operating table or simply becomes trapped as the patient is moved, considerable tension can be exerted on the catheter and its balloon. This has been known to cause serious damage to the posterior urethra and bladder, necessitating surgical repair.

(6) Displacement of intracranial and spinal catheters. Ventricular and spinal drainage systems and epidural catheters have all been known to require replacing as a result of accidents in the course of patient transfer.

Transfer of patients to the operating theatre

In the authors' opinion, transfer of the patients in their beds represents the ideal. There is minimal disturbance, which is advantageous in the already premedicated patient, and it is the most comfortable method. Clearly, height adjustable, easily manoeuvrable beds with good tipping and braking systems and side-guards are ideal.

If patients are sufficiently mobile and cooperative they can transfer themselves across to the theatre trolley or operating table as follows:

(1) The bed and adjacent operating table are adjusted to be at the same height. The brakes are applied on both.

(2) Blankets are removed from the patient leaving one sheet in place.

(3) With nurses then holding the free top and bottom ends of the sheet the patient moves sideways onto the operating table, with help if necessary, remaining covered by the sheet throughout the procedure, and taking his/her time. Patients may be in pain or heavily sedated, and it is essential not to hurry the transfer.

Alternative methods to the above are as follows:

(1) A canvas stretcher and poles can be used to lift the patient from one surface to the other.

(2) Direct lifting of the patient by theatre attendants. In this case the patient is first moved to the edge of the bed nearest to the operating table, and then lifted across by the attendants from the other side of the table. Simultaneous support for the patient's head, chest, pelvis and legs is required for this manoeuvre.

In those hospitals where transfer with ward beds is impracticable a trolley system has to be used. Transfer to the trolley takes place by one of the methods previously described. Privacy from other ward patients can easily be provided by the use of screens or bed curtains. If any further transfer of the patient is likely to be needed using stretcher poles and canvas it is important to remember to insert the canvas at an appropriately early stage, remembering particularly to ensure that the patient's head will be supported.

Trolley-top transfer systems are used in some hospitals. On arrival in the operating theatre transfer zone, the incoming trolley is locked side by side to a trolley base in the clean area. The patient and trolley top are then smoothly moved from one to the other, after ensuring that they are properly locked. Subsequent transfer is usually by stretcher poles and canvas.

Patients with pelvic or lower limb fractures are best transferred from the ward to the operating table in their beds. Anaesthesia is then induced on the bed, prior to placement on the operating table.

Position for postoperative extubation

If, during the course of anaesthesia, the patient has been intubated, there are two aspects of extubation which influence patient position and merit discussion.

(1) Theoretically the lateral position should be advocated for extubation of the patient. The risks of inhaling gastric contents into the lungs have been particularly stressed in Chapter 1. Nevertheless, in the authors' experience the majority of anaesthetists routinely extubate with the patient supine. It is therefore assumed that the following advantages are considered to outweigh the risks.

(a) Theatre attendants are not required to turn and support the patient in the lateral position on a narrow operating table whilst the procedure is carried out.

(b) Coughing and straining on the endotracheal tube, which invariably accompanies movement of the patient when anaesthesia is very light, is avoided.

(c) The use of a laryngoscope and sucker and the application of a face-mask is generally easier in this position.

(d) It is easier to re-intubate in the supine position on the rare occasions that this becomes necessary.

Certain high-risk patients are always managed more safely if extubation is carried out in the lateral position with slight head-down tilt, as when gastric contents are present. The universal availability of good suction apparatus and easily tipped operating tables may reduce the risks of extubation in the supine position. It may also instil a false sense of security.

(2) Extubation may be postponed occasionally until the patient has been transferred to the recovery room. The possible reasons for this decision and the implications for recovery room staff require clarification. Patients so managed usually fall into one of three groups:

(a) Those who have been extremely difficult to intubate so that the anaesthetist wishes to be absolutely sure that emergency re-intubation will not be required.

(b) Those patients awaiting a fuller recovery from the depressant effects of the anaesthetic.

(c) Those patients deemed to require protection of the tracheal airway from soiling by gastric contents, blood or cerebrospinal fluid.

In the last group of patients the endotracheal tube cuff will have been left inflated and therefore it is acceptable and probably preferable to nurse the patient in the supine position. If, however, the cuff has been left deflated, as is likely in the first two groups, then the patient must be nursed in the lateral position.

Instructions for positioning the patient and subsequent management rest only with the anaesthetist, who must remain within the theatre complex and in charge of the patient.

Transfer of the patient from the operating room

Unconscious patients can neither cooperate in the move nor protect themselves from the dangers involved. The hazards outlined earlier in the chapter are therefore particularly pertinent to this phase of patient transfer.

Once extubation has been satisfactorily achieved the patient should be turned into the full lateral position. Transfer from the operation room is generally a reversal of the incoming procedure and will not be discussed in detail. Where the use of stretchers or transfer trolleys is not applicable the unconscious patient may have to be manually lifted or transferred laterally with the use of a 'roller':

Manual transfer

This commonly takes place in a lateral direction but may, on occasion, take place with the bed positioned 'in tandem' to the operating table. In either case the anaesthetist must take responsibility for the head and neck and three other attendants should be positioned to lift chest, pelvis and legs respectively. A direct lateral lift is safer from the patient's point of view as the distance traversed is minimal. A longitudinal transfer may be the better method when maintenance of a particular position is desirable, e.g. following hip replacement surgery (as in Chapter 7).

The roller

This piece of equipment permits lateral transfer of the patient for the least physical effort by theatre staff. It is particularly useful for obese patients. It consists of an oblong metal frame approximately 2 metres long and 0.5 metre wide within which are arranged five longitudinally aligned metal tubes (*Figure 6.12*). They are free to rotate about their long axis and are covered by a firm rubber fabric which slides across the upper and lower surfaces around the two longitudinal boundaries.

Method of use

(1) Before starting the transfer the brakes on both the operating table and adjacent bed or trolley must be firmly secured and their heights adjusted to the same level. They must be as close as possible and any narrow gaps should be bridged by longitudinally placed pillows (*Figure 6.13*).

(2) With the anaesthetist supporting the head and neck, a minimum of two assistants, standing on the operating table side, roll the patient slightly towards themselves (*Figure 6.14*). This can be done most simply by raising the appropriate edge of the underlying canvas stretcher.

(3) The 'roller' is then placed longitudinally beneath the raised canvas stretcher and the patient is lowered back into the supine position. Both feet must be on the roller.

(4) Having finally checked that all drainage tubes, urinary catheters and infusion lines are free to move with the patient, two assistants on the receiving side firmly pull the near edge of the canvas towards themselves, and the patient will glide smoothly from one surface to the other (*Figure 6.15*).

(5) The operating table is then moved away and the patient turned into the full lateral position. The underlying canvas stretcher is removed unless required later (*Figure 6.16*).

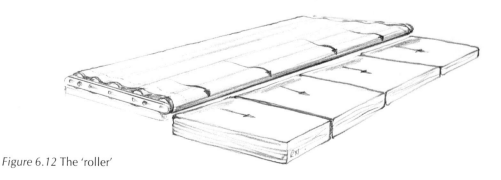

Figure 6.12 The 'roller'

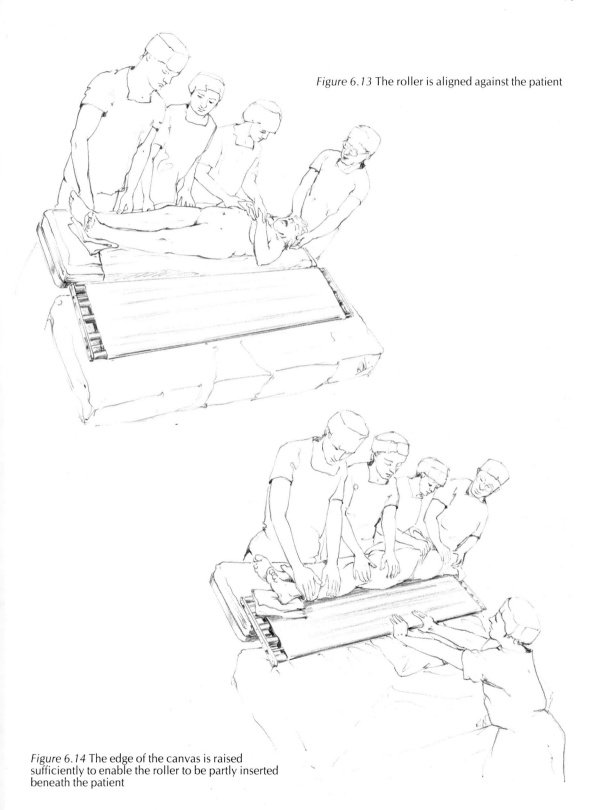

Figure 6.13 The roller is aligned against the patient

Figure 6.14 The edge of the canvas is raised sufficiently to enable the roller to be partly inserted beneath the patient

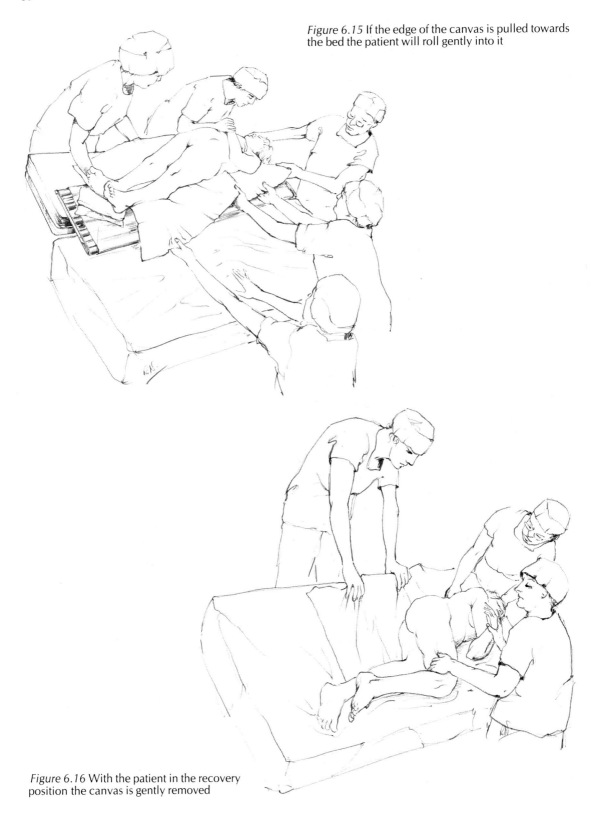

Figure 6.15 If the edge of the canvas is pulled towards the bed the patient will roll gently into it

Figure 6.16 With the patient in the recovery position the canvas is gently removed

In some situations where the stretcher canvas has not been used initially, or where it has become heavily soiled, it may be desirable to move the patient directly on top of the roller. This is quite feasible but generally does not result in such a smooth transfer. It does put the patient's skin at some slight risk of abrasion. In the authors' opinion, the stretcher canvas should be used wherever possible.

Position in the recovery room

Good access to the head-end of the patient is absolutely mandatory in the early recovery period. The bed or trolley must not be positioned against a wall or in any way which might impede this. Bed-head boards should be detachable and not replaced until the patient is safe to leave the recovery area.

Unconscious or semiconscious patients must always be in a position where their airways can be maintained without the risk of aspiration. The posterior part of the tongue must therefore not be allowed to fall back against the pharyngeal wall and the pharynx itself should be dependent (*Figure 6.17*). In practice this means, therefore, that the patient is in the full lateral position with the head-end slightly lowered (*Figure 6.18*).

In the authors' experience and that of Notcutt (1981) many patients are transferred to the recovery room in the supine position and remain so throughout their stay. It may be that the anaesthetists concerned respect the ability of their nursing staff to deal with any of the emergencies which could arise. A high standard

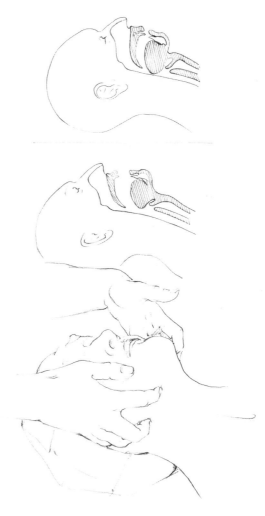

Figure 6.17 In an unconscious patient the posterior part of the tongue may occlude the airway. Pulling the jaw forward, by the angle if necessary, will relieve the obstruction caused by the tongue

Figure 6.18 Postoperative recovery position

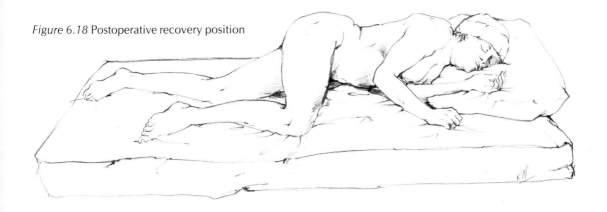

of equipment, suction and tipping trolleys engender a state of false security. It must be emphasized that 20 per cent of all cases of death and serious neurological damage related to anaesthesia have occurred in the immediate recovery period (Green, 1986). Lunn and Mushin (1982) also draw attention to the fact that 17.5 per cent of the anaesthetic deaths they investigated occurred in hospitals with no proper recovery facilities. The recovery period is undoubtedly a hazardous one for the patient and correct lateral positioning may well have prevented some of these tragedies. Nurses in the recovery room should only accept patients into their care in the supine position if they are either already fully awake or if there is some over-riding surgical or medical reason for avoiding the lateral position.

In some instances it may be prudent to retain a patient in the recovery room after the 'immediate recovery phase' (Steward and Volgyesi, 1978) has been completed. Consciousness has been regained and vital functions are stable and can be maintained without assistance. A change in posture then may be appropriate and it is not uncommon for the patient to be placed supine with the back-rest raised to approximately 45 degrees. The generally accepted rationale for this is that diaphragmatic action is less impeded and it has been shown that the functional residual capacity of the lungs increases (Hsu Ho and Hickey, 1976). However, Russell (1981) has studied respiratory function in 19 patients subjected to such changes, at approximately 30 to 60 minutes after the completion of surgery. There was a statistically significant deterioration in arterial oxygenation in most patients when sitting up. The changes in blood levels of oxygen and carbon dioxide can be seen in *Figure 6.19*. Adverse changes in the perfusion of blood through the lungs might be responsible for negating the expected benefits in oxygenation. It would appear from this work that there is no advantage in this change of posture. Should it be deemed necessary for any reason, adequate oxygen should be continuously given and blood gases monitored.

In the future it seems likely that the pressure of increasing workloads on intensive care units will force an expansion in the accepted role of the recovery room. Both cardiac (Aps, Hutter and Williams, 1986) and neurosurgical patients

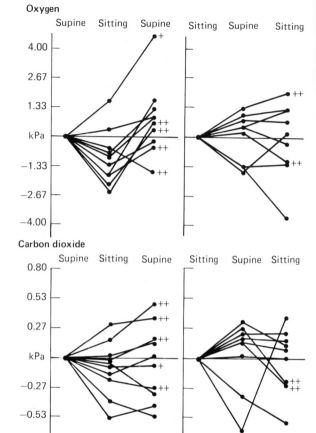

Figure 6.19 Effect of the supine position and sitting up on arterial oxygen and carbon dioxide tensions. The value at the initial position was taken as the baseline. Each point is the average of two measurements taken at 15 and 20 minutes after positioning.
+ = Patient smoking up to nine cigarettes a day.
++ = Patient smoking ten or more cigarettes a day.
NB Sitting is defined as '45° propped up' position.
(From Russell, 1981, reproduced by permission of the author and publishers)

may require admission to such units. Reports detailing some of the postural implications for these specialities have appeared recently:

(1) Chulay and Miller (1984) have studied the effect of back-rest elevation on pulmonary artery and pulmonary capillary wedge pressures in patients within 24 hours of cardiac surgery. Both parameters remained stable when the back-rests were elevated to 20, 30 and 45 degrees and there was no significant difference whether the patients had elevated levels, were

being mechanically ventilated or were receiving vasoactive drugs. They conclude that their results support other studies that pulmonary artery and pulmonary capillary wedge pressures can be measured accurately with the back-rest of the bed elevated to 45 degrees. This has important implications for patient comfort and the saving of nursing time, since former practice was always to take these measurements in the supine position. Rabow, Dwane and Don (1972) measured gas exchange and cardiac output in 12 patients the day after cardiac surgery involving total cardiopulmonary bypass. Measurements taken in the horizontal position were compared with those made with the trunk of the patient flexed at approximately 35 degrees to the horizontal. There was no significant difference in arterial oxygen levels, alveolar to arterial oxygen gradient or cardiac output. The arterial carbon dioxide level decreased slightly but significantly in the head-up position. They concluded that the approximately 35 degree head-up position could be used safely to make patients subjectively more comfortable, but there was no evidence of any improvement in cardiorespiratory parameters.

(2) Neurosurgical patients with raised intracranial pressure are sensitive to changes in body position and to rotation of the head. Mitchell, Ozuna and Lipe (1981) investigated such patients and found that turning from supine to either lateral position or *vice versa* increased the mean intracranial pressure for at least 5 minutes in all patients. Although the increase in most subjects was not to a degree that might have been harmful had it not been prevented by the drainage system, one-third of the patients had increases of more than $20\,cmH_2O$. Head rotation to the right gives a greater and more consistent rise in intracranial pressure than turning to the left. The important conclusion from this study was that although the magnitude of increase in intracranial pressure consequent on repositioning the patient may not always be clinically dangerous it cannot be predicted, from readily available clinical data, which patients are at risk. Monitoring is therefore especially important.

References

Aps, C., Hutter, J. A. and Williams, B. T. (1986) Anaesthetic management and postoperative care of cardiac surgical patients in a general recovery ward. *Anaesthesia,* **41**, 533–537

Chulay, M. and Miller, T. (1984) The effect of backrest elevation on pulmonary artery and pulmonary capillary wedge pressures in patients after cardiac surgery. *Heart and Lung,* **13**, 138–140

Farman, J. V. (1978) The work of the recovery room. *British Journal of Hospital Medicine,* **19**, 606–616

Green, R. A. (1981) The 'butterfly needle'. *The Medical Protection Society Annual Report,* 20

Green, R. A. (1986) A matter of vigilance. *Anaesthesia,* **41**, 129–130

Harvey, D. C. (1983) The reliability of 'butterfly' needles during anaesthesia. *Anaesthesia,* **38**, 1102

Hsu Ho and Hickey, R. F. (1976) Effect of posture on functional residual capacity postoperatively. *Anesthesiology,* **44**, 520–521

Lunn, J. N. and Mushin, W. W. (1982) *Mortality Associated with Anaesthesia.* The Nuffield Provincial Hospitals Trust, London, 21–22

Mitchell, P. H., Ozuna, J. and Lipe, H. P. (1981) Moving the patient in bed: Effects on intracranial pressure. *Nursing Research,* **30**, 212–218

Notcutt, W. G. (1981) Problems in the immediate post-anaesthetic period. *British Journal of Hospital Medicine,* **25**, 646

Rabow, F. I., Dwane, P. and Don, H. (1972) The effect of posture on gas exchange following cardiac surgery. *Canadian Anaesthetists Society Journal,* **19**, 647–650

Russell, W. J. (1981) Position of the patient and respiratory function in the immediate postoperative period. *British Medical Journal,* **283**, 1079–1080

Sale, J. P. (1984) The use of butterflies. *Anaesthesia,* **39**, 294

Steward, D. J. and Volgyesi, G. (1978) Stabilometry: A new tool for the measurement of recovery following general anaesthesia for out-patients. *Canadian Anaesthetists Society Journal,* **25**, 4–6

Tully, J. L., Friedland, G., Baldini, L. M. and Goldmann, D. A. (1981) Complications of intravenous therapy with steel needles and teflon catheters. *American Journal of Medicine,* **70**, 702–706

Chapter seven

Specialized positions

This chapter has been included to give a series of brief descriptions of positions which, although quite commonly used, are of a specialized nature. Positioning is usually carried out by the surgeon or anaesthetist, but in some instances the theatre nurse or technician may be expected to assist. An understanding of the objectives and the hazards is therefore essential. Positions will be discussed under the heading of the relevant surgical specialty:

(1) Ear, nose and throat surgery
(a) The Boyle–Davis gag
(b) Position for microlaryngeal surgery

(2) Orthopaedic surgery – the orthopaedic 'fracture' table

(3) Neurosurgery – application of the 'three-pin head-rest'

(4) Use of the evacuatable mattress

(5) Position in the dental chair

(6) Positioning for cardiopulmonary resuscitation.

Ear, nose and throat surgery

The Boyle–Davis gag

This is used primarily for adenotonsillectomy and occasionally for the surgery of other lesions of the mouth. The surgical requirement is to produce a clear view and the best possible access to an awkwardly sited operative field. It has two components:

(1) a combined mouth gag and tongue depressor (*Figure 7.1*),

(2) a pair of metal rods from which the gag can be suspended (*Figure 7.2*).

Original models were designed before the routine use of endotracheal anaesthesia. These versions, therefore, do not have a central split along the blade (Doughty, 1957), which nowadays houses the endotracheal tube. They are still used either when a nasal endotracheal tube has been preferred or where surgery is only taking place on one side of the mouth. In this case, an oral endotracheal tube is placed along the contralateral margin of the tongue and the blade of the gag is centrally placed as usual. Some obsolete versions may even have an attachment for the pharyngeal insufflation of anaesthetic gases.

Preliminary anaesthetic considerations
(1) Following induction of general anaesthesia, a preformed oral endotracheal tube of the 'Rae' type (*Figure 7.3*) is passed and secured with adhesive tape in the midline of the mouth. This ensures that the first connection to the breathing circuit is not in close proximity to the gag and is therefore less prone to accidental disconnection. The breathing circuit is connected and runs caudally towards an anaesthetic machine situated at the side or end of the operating table. Alternatively, a nasal endotracheal tube is passed, in which case the extended breathing hose is routed up over the forehead and down beneath the table to the anaesthetic machine.

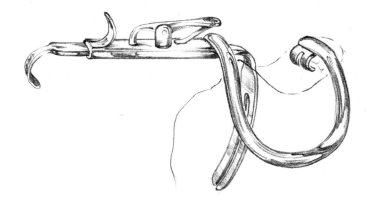

Figure 7.1 Boyle—Davis combined mouth gag and tongue depressor

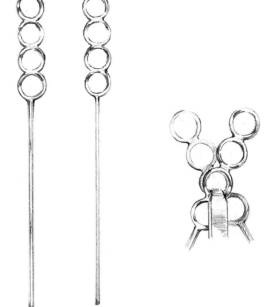

Figure 7.2 Suspension rods for the Boyle—Davis gag

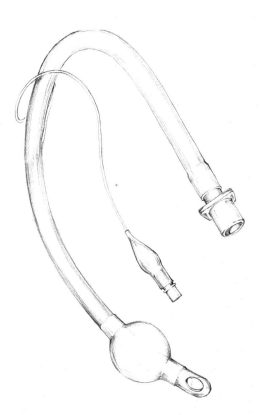

Figure 7.3 The 'Rae' pre-formed oral endotracheal tube

(2) A small firm pad is placed under the shoulders to elevate them slightly.

(3) The pillow is removed and replaced by a head ring in order to allow positioning of the support rods on the adjacent mattress. A metal base plate specially drilled to receive and stabilize the lower ends of these rods may be used if available, but has not been found to be universally satisfactory (*Figure 7.4*).

(4) The patient's eyes must be covered.

The anaesthetist must be vigilant at all stages to ensure that:
(a) Disconnection of the endotracheal tube, or even inadvertent extubation, does not occur as a result of manipulation of the patient's head, particularly when the surgical drapes are being applied.
(b) There is no kinking of the endotracheal tube, particularly if it does not 'match' the split in the gag (Buckley and Bush, 1985), or gets trapped against the teeth.

Figure 7.4 The position for tonsillectomy using Boyle–Davis gag with bipods and base plate. Note the small pad supporting the shoulders

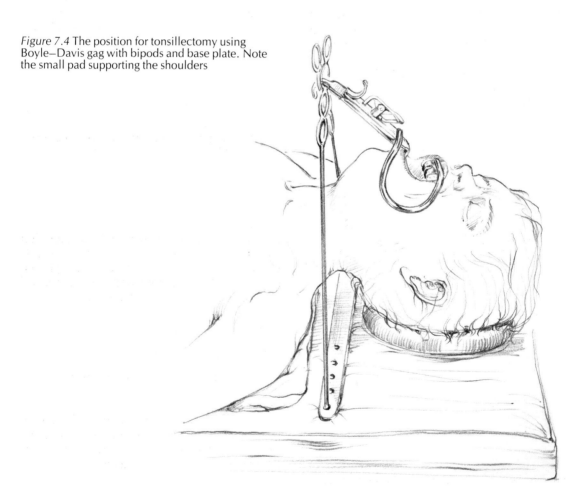

Positioning the gag

(1) The closed gag is inserted over the tongue in the midline until the anterior upper and lower teeth can be comfortably housed in their respective grooves. Care is taken not to crush or bruise the lips or to dislodge any loose teeth or artificial dental caps or crowns.

(2) It is then opened sufficiently to provide the best possible view of the operating field. If the adenoids are to be curetted, it is important that they are removed while the surgeon is still holding the gag (*Figure 7.5*). This ensures that anterior curvature of the cervical spine can be limited. If the head is allowed to become hyperextended whilst this procedure is performed, there is a danger that the curette will go too deep and damage ligaments overlying the anterior surface of the vertebral bodies.

(3) The most appropriate rings on the support rods are then inserted simultaneously under the 'hook' of the gag, and their position is adjusted to raise the head sufficiently to give a good view without actually 'suspending' the patient (*Figure 7.6*). Specially shortened supporting rods are sometimes necessary to prevent this problem in small children.

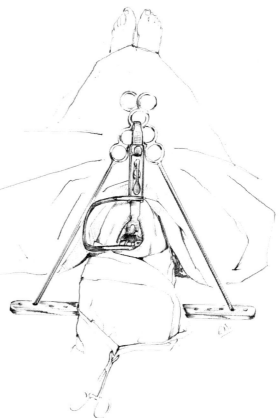

Figure 7.6 Surgeon's view with assembly in position for tonsillectomy

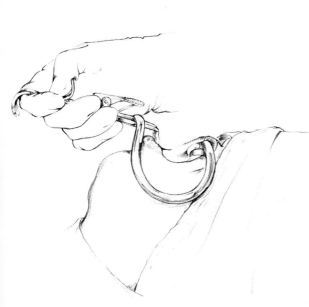

Figure 7.5 Position for adenoidectomy. Surgeon holds the gag to avoid hyperextension of the neck

Risks of use

(1) Care must be taken to avoid hyperextension of the cervical spine. Fortunately, most patients on which it is used are young and supple but older patients with a narrowed spinal canal and osteophyte formation must be managed carefully.

(2) Damage to the teeth.

(3) Dislocation of the mandible.

(4) Airway problems outlined above.

Postoperative positioning

Extubation will be performed following a thorough evacuation of debris or blood from the postnasal space and pharynx. Many anaesthetists always extubate such patients in the lateral position.

Position for microsurgery of the larynx

There are two important 'positional' implications when this procedure is performed under general anaesthesia:

(1) The method of providing an airway down to and through the vocal cords must be absolutely reliable and set up in such a way that it does not become either disconnected or obstructed.

(2) The airway below the surgical field, in addition to remaining patent, should not permit soiling of the lungs by blood secretions or surgical debris.

Fastidious care must be taken whilst setting up the anaesthetic and position of the patient, and throughout surgery it is essential that both the surgical and anaesthetic teams remain mindful that even slight adjustments to position may compromise the airway. Adequate and continuous monitoring of lung ventilation is mandatory and instant correction must be instituted for faults detected.

The main principles of positioning for microsurgery of the larynx are outlined in *Figure 7.7* and the simplest method of providing airway control has been chosen (Keen, Kotak and Ramsden, 1982). Alternative methods using jet-ventilation have also been advocated (Carden and Vest, 1974).

In relation to the technique (*Figure 7.7*) attention must be paid to the following points:

(1) Method of support for head and shoulders.

(2) Protection for the eyes.

(3) Plastic 'guard' on the upper teeth.

(4) Endotracheal tube;
(a) narrow bore size, 5 mm for adult,
(b) passed nasally – sits posteriorly in the larynx, not obstructing the surgeon's view,
(c) high volume, low pressure cuff sited below the vocal cords,
(d) secured by adhesive strapping and Clausen's harness,
(e) breathing circuit away from surgeon,
(f) use of IPPV because of the narrow tube.

Figure 7.7 Positioning for microsurgery of the larynx. See text for description of details

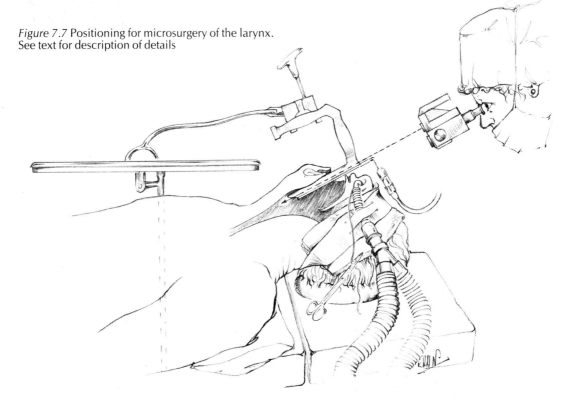

(5) The laryngoscope with the support 'jack'. The latter, although designed to rest on the patient's chest is better positioned on a Mayo table for the following reasons:

(a) It can exert considerable pressure, which is undesirable, either on the chest or, if used with children, on epigastric structures.

(b) It is absolutely vital to be able to see the chest movement because, with the narrow endotracheal tube, inspiration must be seen to be adequate. Expiration, which is passive, and therefore usually much slower, must be completed before the next inspiration is commenced. Failure to allow for this can result in 'progressive chest inflation'. Both the position of the patient and the arrangement of the surgical drapes should take this into account.

When surgery has been completed and spontaneous respiration is judged to be adequate, extubation should be performed with the patient in the supine position. There is always a significant risk of laryngospasm and if this is severe or intractable, re-intubation or even emergency tracheostomy may have to be resorted to. Once the immediate danger of this complication is over, the patient should be turned to the lateral position and transferred to the recovery room.

Positioning patients on an orthopaedic operating table

This is an operating table in which the bottom one-third has been modified along the lines of the original Watson Jones traction table (Wilson, 1982) to facilitate the intra-operative management of patients with a fracture of the femoral neck (*Figure 7.8*). The essential features are:

(1) a vertical padded post to prevent the pelvis moving caudally when traction is applied to the feet;

(2) separate adjustable horizontal extensions to support the legs. The latter are secured by placing each foot in a specially mounted surgical boot.

The patient is usually positioned with the legs apart so that an image intensifier X-ray machine can be used at the operative site.

Management of the patient

(1) The first priority in the pre-operative preparation is to avoid any exacerbation of pain associated with the fracture. The patients are therefore brought to the anaesthetic room in their ward bed and if general anaesthesia is to

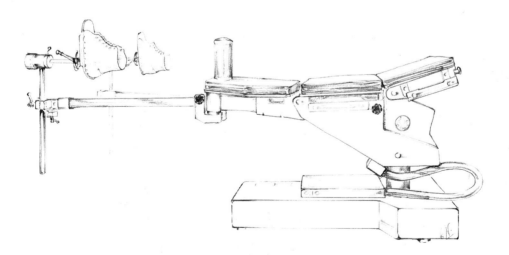

Figure 7.8 Orthopaedic 'traction' table with perineal post and adjustable extensions for securing the legs

be used induction takes place without further transfer. These patients are never so urgent that 'the full stomach' should present a problem, but nevertheless the usual precautions to retain full control of the airway and to cope with unexpected gastric regurgitation must be observed. Patients for epidural or spinal anaesthetic usually need to sit upright whilst this is performed. It is a matter for individual judgement whether the subsequent advantages of these techniques outweigh the discomfort the patient may experience when positioned for the block.

(2) To enhance ease of access, intravenous infusions should be sited on the contralateral arm to the fracture site.

(3) Following induction of anaesthesia and the completion of other anaesthetic preparations, the patient is moved to the operating table. This can be done most satisfactorily by aligning the one with the other 'in tandem' (*Figure 7.9*). The anaesthetist must take responsibility for the head and neck whilst at least three other strong assistants, all arranged on the same side, lift and carry the patient from one to the other.

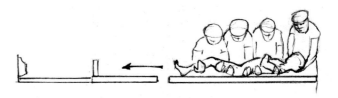

Figure 7.9 Longitudinal transfer of the patient to the fracture table

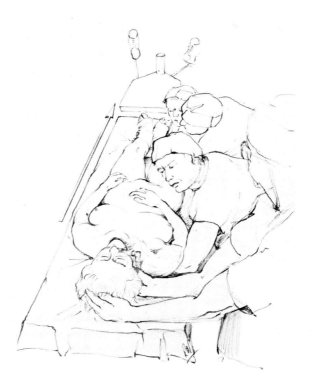

(4) The surgical team are responsible for positioning the lower part of the body and this involves ensuring that the symphysis pubis is in contact with the padded perineal post without damaging the genitalia. It is advised that the post be positioned between the genitalia and the uninjured lower limb in order to minimize the chances of damage to the pudendal nerve (Hofmann, Jones and Schoenvogel, 1982). The patient should be positioned so that the operation site is at the lateral edge of the operating table. Surgical manipulation of the fracture may be required at this stage and following its completion the feet are placed within the boots. The position of the legs is adjusted so that the necessary traction is applied and they are abducted to accommodate the 'C' arm of the image intensifier. Abduction of the affected hip should not exceed 20 or 30 degrees if angulation at the fracture site is to be avoided (Campbell, 1971). The intensifier is positioned before skin preparation and draping of the patient (*Figure 7.10*).

Postoperative management

On completion of surgery, the feet are released and supported, the perineal post is removed, and the patient is then lifted laterally straight into bed. Multiple transfer via trolleys to the patient's bed is undesirable. Care must be taken to ensure that catheters, infusion lines and wound drainage tubes and bottles do not become detached.

Figure 7.10 Position of X-ray image intensifier allowing direct visualization of fracture site in vertical and horizontal axes

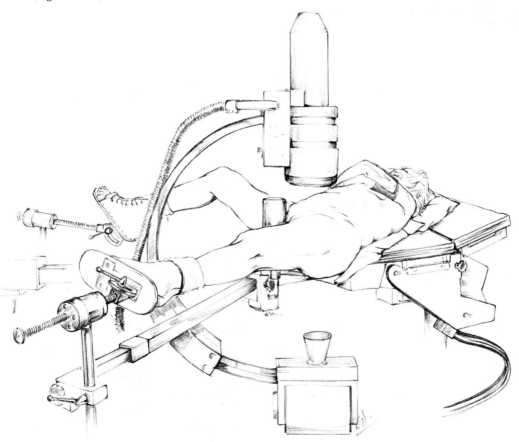

Use of the 'three-pin head-rest' for neurosurgical procedures

These devices serve three important functions:

(1) They provide the absolutely stable skull fixation which is essential for intricate intracranial surgery.

(2) Their position of application can be varied, thus allowing the surgeon a greater freedom of access.

(3) Pressure damage to the skin, occasionally seen when the head is supported by conventional methods, is avoided.

Modern versions of the apparatus are developed from earlier work by De Martel (1931) and Gardner (1935; 1955) (*Figure 7.11*). The original versions were supported by the simple 'adjustable rod' mechanism still commonly used for the 'horseshoe' head-rest. The 'Mayfield system' of support is superior and gives absolute security with an almost infinitely variable selection of positions (*Figure 7.12*). It can be used both with its own design of head-rest or the Gardner version.

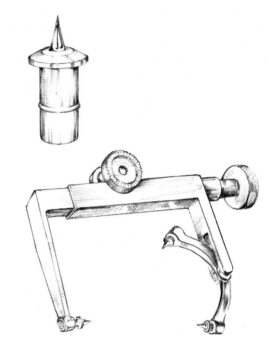

Figure 7.11 The 'three-pin head-rest' or 'skull clamp'

The apparatus

As can be seen in the illustrations, both systems consist of two arms joined by an adjustable cross-member. One of these carries a single pin, whilst its opposite number supports the remaining two pins on a centrally pivoted curved bar. Two types of pin are used, depending on the depth of bony penetration which is required. They are detachable and are retained within their sockets by a spring O-ring.

Application

This is always performed by a member of the surgical team in order to ensure that the position of the pins meets the exact requirements of the surgical procedure and any intra-operative radiography. Areas of the skull known to have relatively thin underlying bone, such as the frontal sinuses or the temporal regions, are usually avoided.

The skin is prepared with the application of an antiseptic solution, but adjacent hair need

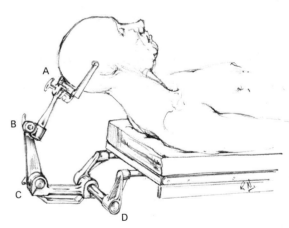

Figure 7.12 The 'Mayfield' system of support for the three-pin head-rest

not be removed. The appropriate (autoclaved) pins are inserted into their sockets and the arms widely separated to accommodate the patient's head. As the two arms of the head-rest are tightened towards one another, the pins penetrate the skin and bite into the outer table of bone. They must always be applied at right-angles to the surface for maximum security. A pressure-sensing gauge is located within the central arm, which measures the force being applied. In paediatric cases 20–30 lb of pressure may be adequate but for adult heads approximately 50 lb is required. It is unwise to put too much reliance on this system. The 'experienced hand' in judging the grip achieved once the pins are firmly located is more valuable. The surgeon should then double-check that the skull is securely clamped within the head-rest before proceeding further.

Finally, the three-pin head-rest is secured to the appropriate attachment on the operating table. The Mayfield (*see Figure 7.12*) system is extremely reliable, adequately variable and simple to use. When the patient is in the supine, prone or lateral position the base unit (D) slides into the conventional cylindrical holders beneath the operating table. When used for patients in the sitting position a special bar attachment is fitted to the lateral rails of the operating table (*Figure 7.13*).

The attachment of the head-rest to the Mayfield system (A) and the first adjustable joint (B) both have ratchet-type interlocking surfaces and are secured by a hand-tightened screw. Care must be taken that cross-threading of the latter does not occur, as it is relatively easy to strip the thread. These are tightened with the head held in the approximately correct position selected by the surgeon, the head is then placed in the exact alignment required and the clutch lever between C and D snapped shut to make the whole system rigid (*Figure 7.12*).

For good operating conditions to ensue, extremes of lateral rotation of the head and neck must be avoided. Similarly, flexion of the head at the atlanto-occipital joint should be the minimum that is acceptable for the proposed operation. It is better to position the patient fully lateral with the head in the 'neutral' position if this is what surgical access demands, rather than to compromise supine positioning by head and neck rotation.

Removal of the head-rest

At the completion of surgery, it is important that anaesthesia is maintained until the head-rest has been removed safely. Any body movement allowed to occur whilst the head is so securely fixed will place a serious stress on the neck muscles and cervical spine and may also cause intracranial congestion. The first step is to disconnect and remove the Mayfield support system from the operating table and replace it by the conventional head-rest. With the head correctly supported on the latter, the three-pin head-rest is released and removed. Care must be taken to avoid scalp lacerations. The resultant punctate scalp lesions are dressed and temporary pressure is applied if any bleeding ensues. This is usually easily controlled and the wounds generally heal quickly.

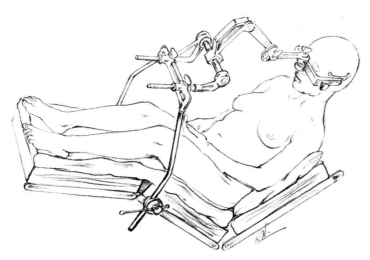

Figure 7.13 The sitting position for neurosurgery using the three-pin head-rest

The role of the evacuatable mattress (Evac M) in positioning patients on the operating table

This has been described by the late Dr J. V. I. Young of the Department of Anaesthetics at The London Hospital. The evacuatable mattress (Evac M), pillow or bag can be regarded as the opposite of an inflatable type. Polystyrene or terylene granules are enclosed in a heavy duty, air tight, flexible plastic container. Air can be sucked out or let in through a stoppered valve or port. When evacuated the consistency changes, it firms up and holds its shape until opened to the atmosphere again (*Figure 7.14*).

Several shapes and sizes (e.g. head support, sacral cushion, trunk support) are supplied by Howmedica, with the trade name 'Vac-Pac', for use on the operating table. Laerdal Medical Ltd produce a full length (approximately 2 metres) example designed for ambulance stretchers, and intended for immobilizing injured patients during transit. The following account is largely concerned with their use in the operating theatre.

Advantages of the evacuatable mattress (Evac M)

(1) *Secure fixation*. The patient can be supported in awkward positions without the necessity for back, pelvic or chest rests and their attendant disadvantages. Furthermore, the conforming nature of the Evac M reduces any tendency to slide if the operation table needs to be tilted steeply.

(2) *Pressure on the skin is evenly and widely distributed*. The Evac M increases the surface area supporting the patient's weight by conforming to body contours. It is more efficient than either sheepskin or gamgee in preventing pressure sores.

(3) *Insulation*. Polystyrene has excellent heat insulating properties. Heat loss by conduction is minimized in skin in contact with an Evac M. When used in conjunction with a space blanket to reduce radiant and convected heat loss, the problem of a significant fall in body temperature in, for instance, long neurosurgical procedures is overcome. This feature is also useful in surgery in infants and young children.

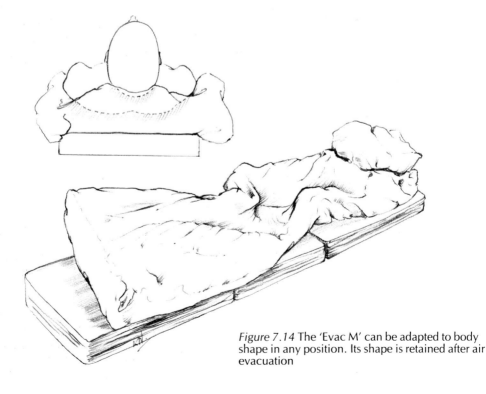

Figure 7.14 The 'Evac M' can be adapted to body shape in any position. Its shape is retained after air evacuation

Disadvantages

(1) *The Evac M is not antistatic.* Although the use of inflammable inhalation anaesthetic agents is declining and debatable, this fact must be noted; polystyrene is a substance particularly prone to attract static charges.

(2) *The stretcher canvas needs to be removed* from beneath the patient since the Evac M is most effective when in direct contact with the skin.

(3) *It is impossible to break or unbreak the operating table* without softening the Evac M; if this manoeuvre is likely to be required during the operation the mattress should not be used.

(4) *The PVC covering is easily torn or punctured.* The commonest leak is due to puncture by surgical towel clips. It is possible to manage a small leak by the use of continuous controlled suction to match it; control is required to keep the suction down to 20–24 mmHg (2.5–5.0 kPa) – uncontrolled strong suction can damage the filling and even squash the patient if persisted with long enough. The puncture can be located when the Evac M is out of use, by blowing it up with air or oxygen and detecting bubbles under water or with a soapy film. Repair kits are available with PVC patches and cement.

(5) *Care must be taken if the Evac M is used directly on top of a metal operating table,* i.e. without the standard rubber mattress intervening. The reason is that it is possible to get the granules distributed unevenly, in such a way that part of the patient may be lying with only two layers of PVC between skin and metal.

Positioning the patient

It has been found that the Evac M is particularly useful for patients positioned in the prone or the lateral positions. In both of these, stability is the prime function. However, it is also useful for prolonged surgery in the supine position where, in addition to its use in the prevention of skin pressure problems, its heat retaining properties are an important added bonus.

The prone position

(1) The face can readily be 'contoured' into the soft Evac M in any position desired. Added protection for the cheek and orbit is advisable in long operations and may be provided by a piece of plastic foam packing. This should be positioned before the Evac M is firmed up.

(2) The Evac M is most useful in allowing the neck to be placed and held in the desired position. This usually means that the shoulders are lifted well up and the head lowered to maintain the natural curvature of the cervical spine. It is often not appreciated how much higher the shoulders have to be than the head in the face-down position to avoid extending the neck – a good guide is the absence of a transverse skin crease at the back of the neck (*Figure 7.15*).

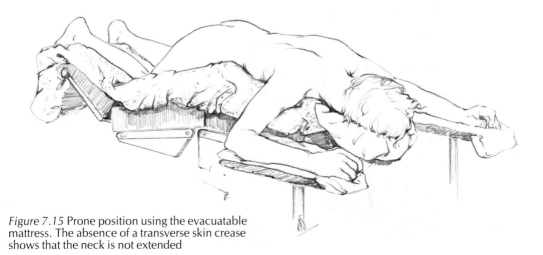

Figure 7.15 Prone position using the evacuatable mattress. The absence of a transverse skin crease shows that the neck is not extended

(3) Undue pressure on the breasts is avoided by the contouring effect without padding. If the arms are placed above the head it helps to have the head of the table angled well down and the top edge of the Evac M about 18 inches (40 cm) beyond the patient's head; by this means the arms may also be secured in the Evac M.

(4) The abdomen needs to be lifted well up away from pressure by raising the pelvis and chest, and then pressing the sides of the Evac M well into the sides of the trunk, particularly at the pelvis and chest, before sucking the air out. This needs to be done with special care before laminectomy. A large pad is sometimes put under the abdomen and removed after hardening the Evac M; this is not always considered to be necessary, as it is thought preferable not to move the patient on a hard Evac M.

The male genitalia may get squashed under the pubic symphysis or thigh in careless positioning. In either sex a urethral catheter should come out straight between the legs with the connecting tube passing over the thigh and attached to it with strapping so that the balloon in the bladder is not dragged on by the weight of a full urine bag.

(5) The legs and feet can be supported in a trough moulded into the Evac M. If a diathermy pad is applied by a circumferential fastening to the thigh it should be done before the final positioning.

The lateral position (*Figure 7.16*)

This position is not easy to assume and has been found to be greatly facilitated by the Evac M. In orthopaedic work such as hip joint replacement, where robust hammering demands a well stabilized patient, it proves almost indispensible once familiarity has been gained.

As an example, the use of it is given in detail:

After anaesthetizing the patient, the diathermy pad is secured on the non-operation thigh. The patient is lifted and turned into the desired position. Normally the trunk, pelvis and lower leg lie in the centre line of the Evac M, which need not be necessarily in the exact midline of the operating table. No canvas or gown is used, the skin being in direct contact. The lower leg and lower hemi-pelvis are secured by rolling up the sides of the soft Evac M and holding firmly, at the same time doing the same along the abdomen, chest and shoulder. The arms come out at right angles; the upper arm may be placed in a forearm rest. This manoeuvre requires up to four pairs of hands with a large patient if it is to be done correctly. When both surgeon and anaesthetist are satisfied, the air is sucked out and the position held secure. The upper (operated) leg should be free to move in any position without disturbing the rest of the patient. It is usually convenient to use the lower arm for the intravenous infusion. It will not become congested unless the patient is obese if the Evac M has been applied carefully. The upper arm can be used for blood pressure recording.

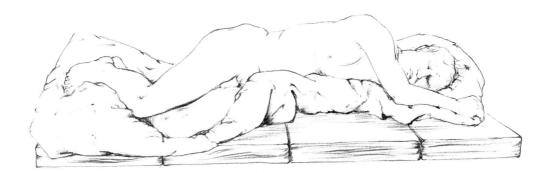

Figure 7.16 Lateral position using the evacuatable mattress. Stability is a valuable asset without using additional support

Paediatric use (*Figure 7.17*)

A suitably sized Evac M may be helpful in the surgery of infants and young children in two ways. Firstly, the part to be operated on can be presented to the surgeon and securely held – especially useful with awkward positions (such as the insertion of ventriculo-atrial or ventriculoperitoneal shunts). Secondly, the insulating properties of polystyrene are most useful in reducing heat loss by conduction. The Evac M should be warmed to body heat before use. With major or long procedures the standard precautions are necessary in addition, including a warm theatre, lotions and irrigating fluids at body temperature, reflective sheeting and heating pad. If the heating pad is under the Evac M the risk of thermal injury to the skin is avoided.

Regional anaesthesia

The Evac M may also be used with advantage in conscious patients undergoing surgery under regional anaesthesia.

Position in the dental chair

Although the incidence is declining, there are still significant numbers of patients submitted to general anaesthesia for dental extractions in the United Kingdom, i.e. in the dentist's surgery or office. They are usually short procedures and are performed without endotracheal intubation. There is a very small, but nonetheless definable, incidence of sudden death associated with the technique reported annually. It has been postulated both that the position of the patient may be a significant factor (Bourne, 1986; Brichard, 1971; Humble, 1971); and that it is insignificant (Tomlin, 1974; Curson and Coplans, 1976; Ayre, 1971).

The dental chair may be placed into one of three configurations; supine, sitting or reclining.

The supine position

Advantages
(1) It is postulated that blood flow to the brain will be better maintained if cardiac output or the blood pressure falls following induction of anaesthesia. Bourne (1957; 1970) drew attention to this and conducted a most vigorous campaign to abandon the use of the then popular sitting position. Vasovagal fainting as a coincidental phenomenon was considered an exacerbating factor in many instances. However, it must be pointed out that fainting can still take place even with the patient fully supine (Verrill and Aellig, 1970). Position alone, therefore, cannot prevent its onset in susceptible patients.

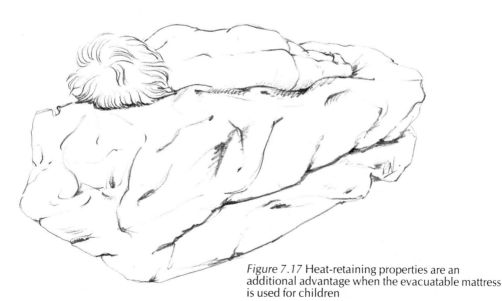

Figure 7.17 Heat-retaining properties are an additional advantage when the evacuatable mattress is used for children

(2) Return to the lateral 'recovery' position can be swiftly and easily achieved and if the surgery is performed on the same trolley that will be used in the recovery area, patient transfer is facilitated.

Contraindications to the supine position

(1) Undue abdominal obesity or advanced pregnancy. Spontaneous respiration may be impaired from pressure on the diaphragm, venous return of blood to the heart may be obstructed by pressure on the inferior vena cava, and increased intragastric pressure may predispose to oesophageal regurgitation.

(2) Hiatus hernia. There is an increased risk of aspiration into the lungs of regurgitated stomach contents. In severe cases, part of the stomach may be incarcerated within the chest and cause respiratory impairment.

(3) Dyspnoeic patients who cannot tolerate the supine position.

Comment

The main advantage of the supine position is that cerebral perfusion may be maintained at a better level should the cardiac output fall, for as long as it takes the more obvious signs of pallor and poor peripheral pulse to become discernible. In the absence of sophisticated cardiovascular monitoring there is a good case for it to be advocated (Blatchley, 1979). It is mandatory to use this position when prolonged operating time is likely, e.g. anticipated difficult extraction or the teaching situation; or where significant cardiac irregularities (common in dentistry) cause a fall in cardiac output.

The sitting position

Advantages

(1) By custom and fairly general agreement, surgical access and ease of extraction has, in the past, been regarded as optimal with the patient sitting up. This argument may not be acceptable to more recently trained dentists, who are accustomed to patients being supine for all procedures.

(2) Breathing is easier in the upright position. Simple measurements with a Wright Respirometer show that when a subject is anaesthetized in the sitting position, with the head tilted slightly backwards and the jaw pushed forward, the patient can maintain normal tidal volumes entirely by nasal breathing, even though the unpacked mouth is wide open (Tomlin and Roberts, 1981).

(3) Experimental work on the positioning of the soft palate has shown that in the upright anaesthetized patient it hangs down to the base of the tongue, whereas in the supine position it falls back, protruding into the airway. There is, therefore, the dual advantage of an improved airway and more efficient sealing off of the pharynx against the inhalation of blood or debris (Tomlin and Roberts, 1981).

(4) Diaphragmatic action is unimpeded in the sitting position.

Contraindications

(1) Small children.

(2) Patients with cardiovascular disease.

(3) Any history of 'fainting'.

(4) Extremely nervous patients.

Comment

Many millions of general anaesthetics have been given without apparent mishap with the patient sitting in the dental chair. This may be due to the inevitable nervous tension, hypoxic gas mixtures or surgical stimulation, causing high circulating adrenaline levels which offset other causes of cardiovascular depression. Tomlin (1974), after a most extensive survey of dental anaesthetic deaths and animal experimentation, concluded that the prime concern of the dental anaesthetist should be to prevent hypoxia occurring. The anaesthetist should choose the technique and position that offers, in his hands, the best protection against this hazard. It would seem prudent, however, to restrict the use of the sitting position to healthy patients having surgery which can be completed in seconds rather than minutes, by dentists and anaesthetists of maturity and skill.

The reclining position

This position was first described by Drummond-Jackson (1969) and later advocated by Levine (1977) as a compromise situation.

Advantages

(1) It is easier for the operator than the full supine position.

(2) There will be minimal impedance to diaphragmatic action.

(3) With the lower limbs raised, gravitational effects will ensure venous return to the pelvis. The negative intrathoracic pressures generated by inspiration will assist.

Contraindications

The pregnant patient.

Comment

Physiologically this position appears to offer little to commend it. Disadvantages to the upper airway are likely to be similar to those of the supine position, respiration may be marginally easier than in the supine position. The cardiovascular advantages are unproven. A major disadvantage for the anaesthetized patient is the virtual impossibility of quickly turning the patient into the lateral recovery position should an emergency arise which necessitates this.

All patients, irrespective of initial position, should be turned into the lateral recovery position, with the dental chair horizontal, as soon as the extractions are completed.

Conclusions

Reduced to the simplest terms, anaesthetized dental patients are at serious risk from either:

(1) a sudden, acute cardiovascular problem, e.g. an arrhythmia with poor cardiac output (Ryder, 1970), or a vasovagal attack which, if not detected, will cause cerebral hypoxia;

(2) neglected respiratory obstruction occurring either during the anaesthetic or the recovery period, ultimately causing hypoxia with secondary cardiovascular and cerebral effects.

An awareness of the possible causes of these problems and continuous monitoring for them make it essential that this work is only carried out by highly skilled and trained personnel. The supine position is, on balance, likely to be the safer one. However, there may still be occasions where the sitting position might be indicated.

Positioning the patient requiring cardiopulmonary resuscitation in the peri-operative period

The details of management are well outside the scope of this book, especially as experienced resuscitators will be in the vicinity and the necessary equipment will be to hand. Comments will be confined strictly to aspects of patient position which may influence the outcome of the procedure.

(1) Tip the operating table or trolley into approximately 15 degrees of head-down tilt. (Alternatively, the patient can remain supine and the legs be raised.) This will be sufficient to enhance venous return to the heart, without causing too much cerebral congestion. It will also increase the chances of successful placement of centrally inserted venous access lines should these be necessary later. On those rare occasions where collapse occurs in a patient with known high central venous pressure the horizontal position should be retained. Steep Trendelenburg is contraindicated as discussed elsewhere.

(2) Place the patient in the supine position. There is no way that effective cardiopulmonary resuscitation can be performed with the patient sitting or prone, and even in the lateral position it will be difficult, unless the surgeon has direct manual access to the heart. If the patient is not already on the relatively firm surface of an operating table or recovery trolley, a board must be placed under the patient, across the full width of the bed, extending from the waist to the shoulder (Adult Advanced Cardiac Life Support, *Journal of the American Medical Association*, 1986) so that effective external cardiac massage can be performed. Never position the head higher than the thorax since even perfectly performed chest compression will not then be able to produce adequate blood flow to the brain. (Adult Basic Life Support, *Journal of the American Medical Association*, 1986). As stated in Chapter 3 a pregnant patient with large uterus must also have a wedge or sandbag placed under the *right* buttock to produce lateral tilt.

In patients where a simple vasovagal attack is suspected (and this can occur even in the supine position) the patient's legs *must* be well elevated. In this condition there is marked vasodilatation of peripheral muscle capillary beds and simple 10 degree tilt may be ineffective. Elevation of the arms may also enhance venous return.

External defibrillation of the heart

Three 'positional' points must be emphasized.

(1) The paddles or electrodes are applied to the chest (Chamberlain, 1986) (*Figure 7.18*).

(2) No part of the patient must be positioned so that it is in contact with the metal of the operating table or trolley, or contact burns may result.

(3) All attendants must stand well clear of the patient when defibrillation is taking place.

Internal cardiac massage

This will necessitate a further change of position. The patient will have to be rolled forwards to a 45 degree right lateral position and stabilized with sandbags or pillows beneath the left shoulder and hip. A surgical incision can then be made in any lower intercostal space, from the edge of the sternum right around the chest wall to the posterior axillary line.

Neonatal resuscitation

The principles of resuscitation are as for adults, but with one major exception, and that is the provision of an external heating source. Even in environments of 20–24°C the core temperature of an asphyxiated wet baby can drop by 5°C in as many minutes. It is essential that an overhead heater with an output of 300–500 watts be mounted about 1 metre above the resuscitation platform (Milner, 1986). Commercially available neonatal resuscitation trolleys incorporate these devices and the patient should always be positioned beneath one.

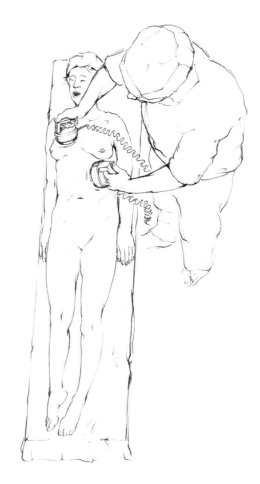

Figure 7.18 The operator applying the electrodes must be positioned well clear of any contact with the patient and the operating table

References

Ayre, P. (1971) Deaths with dental anaesthetics. *Anaesthesia*, **26**, 105–106

Blatchley, D. (1979) The case for the horizontal posture. *Society for the Advancement of Anaesthesia in Dentistry Digest*, **4**(i), 8–9

Bourne, J. G. (1957) Fainting and cerebral damage: a danger in patients kept upright during dental gas anaesthesia and after surgical operations. *Lancet*, **ii**, 499–505

Bourne, J. G. (1970) Deaths with dental anaesthetics. *Anaesthesia*, **25**, 473–481

Bourne, J. G. (1986) Deaths and posture in the dental chair: a 30 year perspective. *Today's Anaesthetist*, **1**(**iv**), 29–33

Brichard, G. (1971) Deaths with dental anaesthetics. *Anaesthesia*, **26**, 106–107

Buckley, P. M. and Bush, G. H. (1985) Split blade tongue retractor. *Anaesthesia*, **40**, 303

Campbell's Operative Orthopaedics (1971) 5th Edn, Vol. i, p. 576. Edited by A. H. Cranshaw. C. V. Mosby, St. Louis

Carden, E. and Vest, H. R. (1974) Further advances in anesthetic techniques for microlaryngeal surgery. *Anesthesia and Analgesia Current Researches*, **53**, 584–587

Chamberlain, D. (1986) ABC of resuscitation (ventricular fibrillation). *British Medical Journal*, **292**, 1068–1070

Curzon, I. and Coplans, M. (1976) Effect of posture on dental anaesthetic mortality. *British Medical Journal*, **ii**, 958

De Martel, T. (1931) Surgical treatment of cerebral tumours. Technical considerations. *Surgery, Gynecology and Obstetrics*, **52**, 381–385

Doughty, A. (1957) A modification of the tongue plate of the Boyle–Davis gag. *Lancet*, **i**, 1074

Drummond-Jackson, S. L. (1969) Intravenous anaesthesia. *Society for the Advancement of Anaesthesia in Dentistry*, London

Gardner, W. J. (1935) Intracranial operations in the sitting position. *Annals of Surgery*, **101**, 138–145

Gardner, W. J. (1955) A neurosurgical chair. *Journal of Neurosurgery*, **12**, 81–88

Hoffman, A., Jones, R. E. and Schoenvogel, R. (1982) Pudendal-nerve neuropraxia as a result of traction on the fracture table. A report of four cases. *Journal of Bone and Joint Surgery*, **64A**, 136–138

Humble, R. M. (1971) Deaths with dental anaesthetics. *Anaesthesia*, **26**, 107–108

Journal of the American Medical Association (1986) Standards and Guidelines for Cardiopulmonary Resuscitation (CPR) and Emergency Cardiac Care (EEC), Multi-author report. **255**, 2905–2989. Adult Advanced Cardiac Life Support, **255**, 2936. Adult Basic Life Support, **255**, 2915

Keen, R. I., Kotak, P. K. and Ramsden, R. T. (1982) Anaesthesia for microsurgery of the larynx. *Annals of the Royal College of Surgeons of England*, **64**, 111–113

Levine, H. A. (1977) Supine or recline. *Anaesthesia Progress*, **24**(**3**), 94–95

Milner, A. D. (1986) ABC of resuscitation. Resuscitation at birth. *British Medical Journal*, **292**, 1657–1659

Ryder, W. (1970) The electrocardiogram in dental anaesthesia. *Anaesthesia*, **25**, 46–62

Tomlin, P. J. (1974) Death in outpatient dental practice. *Anaesthesia*, **29**, 551–570

Tomlin, P. J. and Roberts, J. F. (1981) The airway in the upright anaesthetised patient. *British Dental Journal*, **150**, 312–314

Verrill, P. J. and Aellig, W. H. (1970) Vaso-vagal faint in the supine position. *British Medical Journal*, **4**, 348

Wilson, J. N. (Editor) (1982) *Fractures and Joint Injuries*, 6th edn, Vol. 2, p. 937. Churchill Livingstone, Edinburgh, Melbourne, London and New York

Chapter eight

Physiological effects of posture in the anaesthetized patient

The aim of this chapter will be to answer, as simply as possible, the question, 'How may positioning a patient on the operating table affect the function of major body systems?' As in the foregoing chapters each position will be dealt with separately and discussion will be centred primarily on the cardiovascular and respiratory systems.

The normal human has a complicated but well integrated arrangement of reflex autonomic feedback mechanisms which ensure that an adequately oxygenated blood flow is maintained to all parts of the body irrespective of posture. Unfortunately, these cannot be relied upon to function correctly when the patient is under the influence of potent anaesthetic drugs. Furthermore, information gleaned from research on awake or normally sleeping patients is of limited value in predicting the responses of the anaesthetized patient.

The supine position

From a physiological point of view, this is the one which causes the least overall upset of normal physiology.

Effects on the respiratory system

(1) During spontaneous respiration in either an awake or an anaesthetized patient the dependent (i.e. posterior) part of *the diaphragm* moves more than the anterior part. This is despite having to work against the weight of the underlying abdominal viscera. Clearly, the latter obstruction will be worse in obese

patients or those who have abdominal distension from any cause. As soon as drugs are given to paralyse the patient the resting position of the diaphragm rises slightly. Furthermore, when intermittent positive pressure ventilation (IPPV) is then instituted, it is the non-dependent (i.e. anterior) parts of the diaphragm which undergo the greatest displacement (i.e. where opposing abdominal forces are least) (Froese and Bryan, 1974) (*Figure 8.1*).

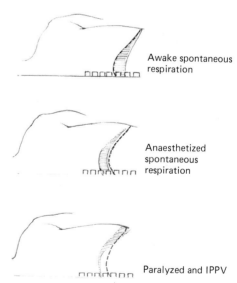

Awake spontaneous respiration

Anaesthetized spontaneous respiration

Paralyzed and IPPV

Figure 8.1 Diaphragm position and displacement during tidal breathing. The dashed line denotes the control functional residual capacity position of the diaphragm. The cross-hatched area represents the diaphragmatic excursion during tidal breathing. (After Froese and Bryan, 1974, reproduced by permission of the authors and publisher)

(2) *The volume of the lungs* is decreased because the abdominal contents push the diaphragm upwards. The effects on that part of the lungs primarily responsible for gaseous exchange (the functional residual capacity, FRC) can be seen in *Table 8.1* (Coonan and Hope, 1983). In the supine position it is reduced by 24 per cent in the conscious patient and by 44 per cent in the anaesthetized state.

(3) *Distribution of inspired gases to functional lung tissue* is altered. This is because the patient's posture and anaesthesia alter both the flow into the lungs and the mechanics of the chest wall and diaphragm. This altered distribution of inspired gases upsets the normal balance between the flow of gas to the alveoli and the corresponding flow of blood through the adjacent capillaries so that, in the final analysis, less oxygen is absorbed (*Figure 8.2*).

Table 8.1 Effect of change in patient's position on functional residual capacity

	Erect		Supine		Prone	Lateral
Conscious	Anaesthetized paralysed	Conscious	Anaesthetized paralysed			
Control value	Reduced by 3%	Reduced by 24%	Reduced by 44%	Reduced by 12%	Increased in dependent lung
						Reduced in uppermost lung

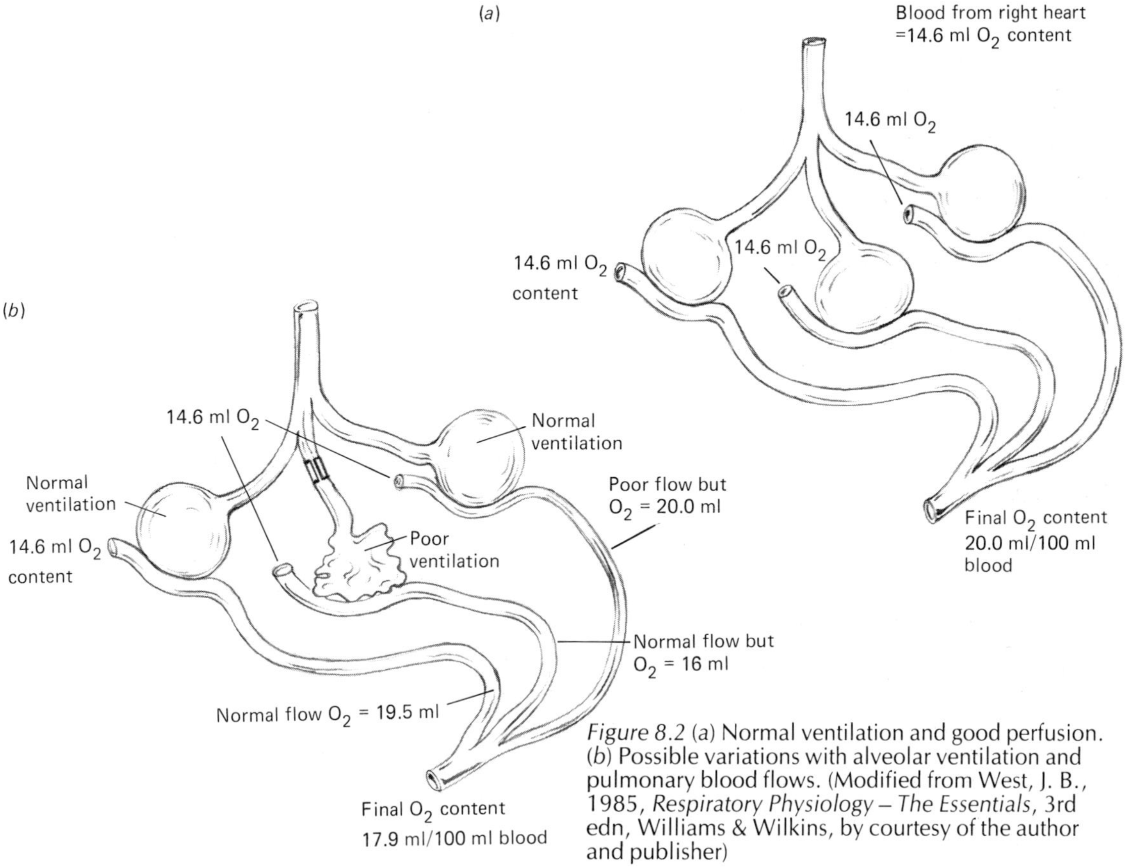

Figure 8.2 (a) Normal ventilation and good perfusion. (b) Possible variations with alveolar ventilation and pulmonary blood flows. (Modified from West, J. B., 1985, *Respiratory Physiology – The Essentials*, 3rd edn, Williams & Wilkins, by courtesy of the author and publisher)

(4) *The volume and distribution of blood flow* through the pulmonary circulation also changes. There is an increase in flow consequent upon the enhanced return of blood to the right side of the heart. The three zones of 'poor', 'intermediate' and 'good' pulmonary blood flow seen from apical to basal areas of the lung in the erect position change through 90 degrees to an anteroposterior axis (West, 1974) (*Figure 8.3*). This to some extent improves the homogeneity of distribution of pulmonary blood volume. Nonetheless, due to the altered distribution of inspired gases referred to above (3) there will be some upset of ventilation/perfusion performance. It is difficult to quantify this effect and often the overall result is linked more to the pre-operative state of health of the patient's lungs rather than to these factors.

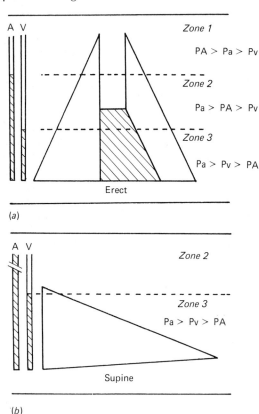

(a)

(b)

Figure 8.3 (a) Schematic diagram of the human heart and lungs in the erect position, showing the three zones postulated by West (1974). (b) Schematic diagram of the human lung in the supine position, showing the preponderance of the Zone 3 effect. (After Coonan and Hope, 1983, reproduced by permission of the authors and publishers)

Effects on the cardiovascular system

This change from the 'normal' erect posture alters the hydrostatic pressures in the veins of the body with consequences for both the systemic and pulmonary circulations. Gravity no longer impedes venous flow from the lower half of the body and there is increased venous return to the right side of the heart. Pulmonary blood flow initially increases as does the output from the left ventricle and, in order to accommodate this, the peripheral resistance falls slightly. Passive hydrostatic effects on the arterial system itself are of little consequence and are easily obscured by active changes in the cardiac output and peripheral resistance. However, it is worth noting that *pressure* at any point in the vascular system is affected by the gravitational forces acting on it. There is a 2 mmHg change in blood pressure for every 2.5 cm of vertical height. This means that with a patient in an erect position the pressure in the cerebral arteries will normally be 25 mmHg less than the pressure measured at heart level, whilst at the feet it will be approximately 115 mmHg higher. Placing the patient in the supine position evens out these differences in arterial blood pressure because hydrostatic forces are always exerted parallel to and in the direction of gravitational pull irrespective of the position of the body.

Plethysmographic studies have shown that the flow of blood through the different organs and peripheral tissues of the body is continuously fluctuating. When a person assumes the supine position and lies immobile, these fluctuations progressively diminish until after about 1 hour they disappear. It is then very difficult for the subject to remain immobile, but if this is achieved, peripheral blood flow further diminishes. In the anaesthetized supine patient an initial increase in peripheral blood flow is followed by a similar fall off of spontaneous volume fluctuations which do not reappear until anaesthesia is terminated and the patient begins to react and move about (Coonan and Hope, 1983).

Summary of cardiorespiratory effects of the supine position

In the spontaneously breathing patient respiration depression by drugs, alterations in pulmonary functioning volumes and changes in blood flow all conspire to reduce the efficiency of oxygen uptake. If IPPV is substituted for spontaneous breathing it may have an adverse effect on cardiac output and, whilst improving the equality of gas distribution, may not always completely improve the ventilation perfusion mismatch.

To some extent the combined disadvantages of general anaesthesia and the supine position are probably ameliorated by the improvement in venous return to the heart and the reduction in cardiac workload required in this position.

The head-down positions

In practice, these are variations of the supine position and exaggeration of the physiological effects described above is to be expected.

Effects on the respiratory system

Conscious volunteers and awake, spontaneously breathing patients frequently find this position intolerable. This is usually due to symptoms of respiratory discomfort or difficulty. Theoretically, respiration can be affected in three ways. Firstly, the weight of the abdominal viscera may impair diaphragmatic movement; secondly, the functioning lung volumes may be reduced by the raised diaphragm and thirdly, gravity may alter the pulmonary circulation. Various reports can be found to support these concepts (Altschule and Zamcheck, 1942; Case and Stiles, 1946; Reed and Wood, 1970). In view of these findings it has been postulated generally that IPPV is mandatory for most patients under general anaesthesia in the Trendelenburg position. However, Scott, Lees and Taylor (1966) have shown that this rule need not be absolute. They investigated arterial blood gas values, ventilation volumes and rates in six healthy young patients under a light general anaesthetic technique allowed to breathe spontaneously in a 35 degree head-down tilted position. Contrary to expectation there was little or no effect on overall respiratory function. In an explanation for this they postulated that the diaphragm, which is able to move very high volumes of air during exercise, is quite capable of the very small extra effort required to compensate for the adverse effects of the head-down position. It must be emphasized that their findings may not be applicable to patients with coincidental cardiorespiratory disease or those having laparoscopic procedures in which ventilation can be embarrassed by intraperitoneal insufflation of carbon dioxide.

Effects on the cardiovascular system

The effects on the cardiovascular system are more complex than is at first apparent.

(1) Theoretically one might expect improved venous return of blood to the heart to increase atrial filling pressure and hence increase cardiac output. However, work carried out in the 1950s (Wilkins, Bradley and Friedland, 1950) on normal patients (albeit with less sophisticated apparatus than is now available), showed no significant haemodynamic benefit. Work on shocked patients in the 1960s (Taylor and Weil, 1967) reached the same conclusions. Sibbald *et al.* (1979) with modern invasive cardiovascular investigative techniques, have monitored the responses to 15–20 degree head-down tilt in 61 normotensive and 15 hypotensive patients with acute cardiac illness or sepsis. In the normotensive patients the preload to the right and left ventricles was increased with a slight increase in cardiac output, but systemic vascular resistance decreased, so that there was no change in mean arterial blood pressure. In the hypotensive patients there was no increase in preload, a slightly increased afterload and a fall in cardiac output.

Similarly, animal studies (Weil and Whigham, 1965; Guntheroth, Abel and Mullins, 1964) have shown that all forms of 'shock' are made worse by the head-down position.

It seems likely that when patients are tipped head-down, the central baroreceptor sensors interpret the increased intravascular pressures at these sites as being generally representative of the total haemodynamic state and respond with an inappropriate fall of systemic vascular resistance. The 'blood pressure' therefore does not rise in the expected manner. A further explanation of failure to improve the shocked patients is that in this condition there may be extensive splanchnic pooling of blood due to localized spasm of the hepatic venous system

(Weil *et al.*, 1956). This will not be corrected by the influence of gravity.

It would appear then, particularly from Sibbald's work, that there is no longer any justification for the time-honoured and continued use of head-down positions in the first aid management of the shocked patient. Simply raising the legs, with the body recumbent, will achieve as much as can be attained in this way.

With very steep tilt, rarely encountered in clinical practice nowadays, (75 degrees) there is a significant decrease in the right atrial filling pressure due to drainage of blood from the heart to the veins of the head and neck (Wilkins, Bradley and Friedland, 1950).

(2) Cerebral blood flow in normal subjects has been shown to decrease by 14 per cent (Shenkin *et al.*, 1949) but does not do so in patients with increased intracranial pressure on short periods of observation. Coonan and Hope (1983) could find no reports of a beneficial effect of the head-down position on cerebral blood flow.

Effects on the eye

Table-tilting experiments by Tarkkanen and Leikola (1967) in which the subjects were varied from 0 to 70 degrees from the horizontal have shown significant elevations of intra-ocular pressure. The amount varies approximately with the sine of the angle that the subject makes with the horizon. From sensitive electrical measurements of optic nerve function made by Friberg and Sandborn (1985) in subjects who volunteered to be completely inverted, it can be concluded that the direct effects of the raised intra-ocular pressure are more important than the increase in intra-ocular perfusion resulting from maintenance of this position. It follows, that steep head-down tilting for any length of time may result in damage to the eye and this will be particularly pertinent in patients already suffering from glaucoma.

The prone position

There are surprisingly little meaningful data published on the cardiorespiratory changes observed in anaesthetized patients in the prone position.

Effect on the respiratory system

Provided that the patient is well supported so that there is no pressure on the abdominal viscera the decrease in functional residual capacity in the prone position is minimal and certainly less than that in either the supine or lateral positions (*Table 8.1*). Gravitational forces obviously play an important role. Although some aspects of lung function have been shown to improve when conscious patients in respiratory failure are turned from the supine to the prone position (Piehl and Brown, 1976; Douglas *et al.*, 1977), the same has not been shown to be the case for healthy patients under general anaesthesia (Stone and Khambatta, 1978).

Effects on the cardiovascular system

Providing there is no obstruction to venous flow resulting from the positioning technique the physiological cardiovascular changes will be broadly in line with those already described for the supine position. In practice, clinically apparent deterioration in cardiac output frequently accompanies the actual positioning manoeuvres and great care must be taken in the immediate post-positioning phase to monitor the cardiovascular system carefully.

Summary of effects of the prone position

Theoretically the cardiovascular and respiratory parameters should be little affected by this position. Unfortunately, coincident medical pathology and the difficulty encountered in easily positioning the obese or awkwardly shaped patient can cause much greater disturbance of cardiovascular system than might be anticipated.

The lateral position

The effects on the respiratory and cardiovascular systems are interrelated and complex and are often compounded not only by the anaesthetic but also by surgery within the thorax.

Effects on the respiratory system

(1) As in the supine position, the weight of the

abdominal contents is transmitted to the lung; in the lateral position the more dependent lung is subjected to further compression by the weight of the heart and great vessels. This leads to a loss of lung volume, particularly where these compressive forces are greatest. Although the total loss of functional residual capacity is slightly less than that found in the supine position it is unevenly distributed: FRC in the dependent lung decreases considerably, while it increases in the upper lung (Rehder and Sessler, 1973).

(2) The distribution of the inspired gas is also altered. The upper lung is favoured in some patients following induction of anaesthesia with spontaneous respiration and in almost all patients if IPPV is used (Rehder et al., 1972) (*Figure 8.4*).

Spontaneous ventilation

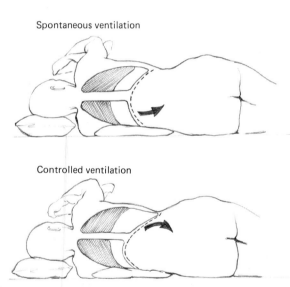

Controlled ventilation

Figure 8.4 Unequal ventilation of the lungs when the patient is in the lateral position

(3) Pulmonary blood flow in the dependent lung depends on the pressure difference between the pulmonary arteries and veins, whereas in the upper lung it depends on the difference between pulmonary artery pressure and the pressure in the airways of that lung (*Figure 8.5*) (because pulmonary venous pressure in the upper lung is very low and is less than the pressure in the alveoli). Several studies have shown a redistribution of pulmonary blood flow

to the most dependent lung regions under conditions of artificial ventilation with or without anaesthesia, and it is probably related to the magnitude of the airway pressure diminishing pulmonary blood flow through the upper lung. This is important, as the redistribution of pulmonary blood flow will generally be unmatched by ventilation, and oxygenation of the patient can be seriously impaired (Denlinger, Kallos and Marshall, 1972; Chevrolet et al., 1978). Furthermore, if fluid volume overload occurs for any reason, it may result in unilateral pulmonary oedema affecting the dependent lung (Snoy and Woodside, 1984).

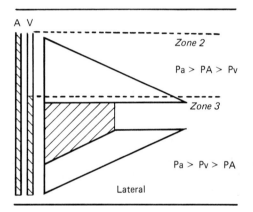

Figure 8.5 Schematic diagram of the human lung in the lateral position, showing the preponderance of the Zone 3 effect. (After Coonan and Hope, 1983, reproduced by permission of the authors and publishers)

Effects on the cardiovascular system

The gravitational effects on the systemic side of the cardiovascular system are similar to, but of lesser magnitude than those described for the supine position. As with the prone position, venous obstruction can be a major factor and impair return of blood to the heart. Lateral positions with the use of a kidney rest may kink major intra-abdominal veins and no longer have a place. Lateral rotation of the neck or extremes of flexion or extension may seriously impede jugular venous drainage or the vertebral arterial supply. This is particularly important when intracranial surgery is performed in the lateral position.

Summary of the cardiorespiratory effects of the lateral position and anaesthesia

In the spontaneously breathing patient the inequalities between lung blood flow and ventilation are not so marked and the physiological upset is not great. Unfortunately, nowadays, the majority of patients having surgery in the lateral position require IPPV for a variety of important reasons. When this is instituted ventilation is favoured to the upper lung and, unless measures to improve oxygenation are taken, there will almost certainly be a deterioration in pulmonary performance.

The sitting position

The controversy over the use of this position has been dealt with in Chapter 7. Although of some relevance to the latter, the physiological considerations detailed below are of greater importance during its use for neurosurgical procedures.

Effects on the respiratory system

(1) Providing the patient is breathing spontaneously the erect position should produce the very least impairment of ventilatory function. Abdominal contents are displaced towards the pelvis so that there is minimal obstruction to diaphragmatic action and there should be no restriction to the anterior expansion of the chest wall produced by other inspiratory muscles.

(2) Because the upright posture helps to hold the alveoli open, the functioning volumes of the lung are less affected during anaesthesia than they are in other positions. This helps to ensure that a high proportion of the blood perfusing the lungs takes part in gas exchange. If these lung volumes were to be adversely affected by the patient's position a greater proportion of the lung blood flow would pass to the systemic side of the circulation without acquiring oxygen. This 'shunted' blood, when mixed in the left side of the heart with well oxygenated blood, reduces the total final oxygen content (*Figure 8.6*).

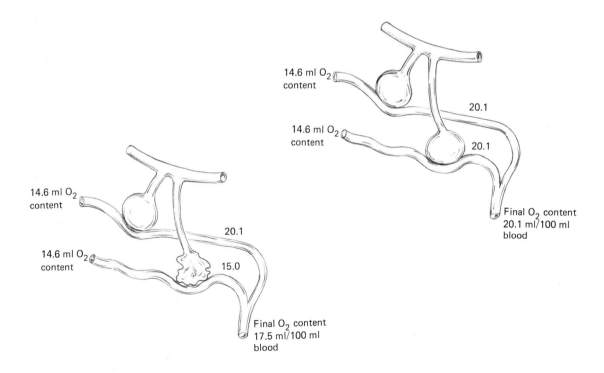

Figure 8.6 Adverse effect of alveolar collapse on oxygenation of pulmonary blood flow

Effects on the cardiovascular system

When an anaesthetized patient is changed from the supine to the erect position blood is transferred from the upper to the lower part of the body. The magnitude of the shift will depend on the exact 'style' of sitting position adopted. Nowadays, the full sitting position with vertical spine and dependent legs is probably rarely used. Clearly, the gravitational effects will be less in those modifications in which the legs and thighs are flexed and feet are at the level of the heart. Dalrymple, MacGowan and Macleod (1979) investigated cardiorespiratory effects in a group of anaesthetized patients using a standard neurolept-type anaesthetic technique. On changing from supine to sitting position heart rate and mean arterial blood pressure were little altered, but a rise of around 50 per cent was necessary in the systemic vascular resistance to compensate for considerable falls in the cardiac output and stroke volume. They concluded that it should not be assumed that a patient who remains normotensive in the sitting position has an adequate circulatory status. Marshall, Bedford and Miller (1983) give data for changes observed with four different anaesthetic techniques and were also able to start their measurements prior to induction of anaesthesia. The cardiovascular effects of sitting the patient up while still conscious are summarized in *Table 8.2*. They are similar to data obtained from healthy normovolaemic volunteers, except that the patients tended to increase their systemic arterial pressure by approximately 11 per cent without a change in cardiac output, and the healthy volunteers maintained a constant blood pressure but their cardiac output fell by 10 per cent. Systemic vascular resistance increased by 10–12 per cent in both groups. Three of the

Table 8.2 Conscious supine to seated position (patients)

Heart rate	+12%
Mean systemic arterial pressure	+11%
Systemic volume indices	+12%
Stroke volume indices	−11%
Pulmonary capillary wedge pressure	−22%
Right atrial pressure	No change
Pulmonary artery pressure	No change
Cardiac index	No change

(From Marshall, Bedford and Miller, 1983)

four anaesthetic techniques discussed were associated with falls in cardiac output around 20–25 per cent and stroke volume index of 25–33 per cent. Systemic arterial pressures fell by 22–27 per cent. The induction of general anaesthesia was more likely to result in a depressed cardiovascular status than was the process of placing the patient into the seated position. There were slight increases in systemic vascular resistance with positioning which was usually enhanced by surgical stimulation. However, the increases were not so marked as noted by Dalrymple and colleagues. The fourth anaesthetic technique (morphine–nitrous oxide) appeared to result in the least impairment of haemodynamic conditions. During induction of anaesthesia the only change was a 20 per cent reduction in stroke volume index, but on positioning the patient cardiac output fell by 25 per cent. This was not improved by surgical stimulation although the latter resulted in a 15 per cent increase in systemic arterial pressure and a 62 per cent in systemic vascular resistance. Cerebral arterial pressure was best protected by this technique since it was maintained at or above control levels during both placement in the seated position and surgery.

Although the healthy patient may well be able to tolerate the haemodynamic changes described, care must be taken in subjecting patients with known cardiovascular impairment to the risks involved. Similarly, patients suffering from reduced blood volume from any cause, or electrolyte and fluid imbalance, may be unable to compensate satisfactorily.

If, after assuming the erect position, there is evidence of low blood pressure accompanied by a slow heart rate, it must be assumed that the phase II cardiovascular changes of vasovagal syncopy are occurring. This highly dangerous situation can only be reversed by tilting the patient supine with the feet elevated (Epstein, Stampfer and Beisser, 1968).

From studies on patients undergoing chemotherapy for cerebral tumours it seems likely that patients anaesthetized in the sitting position have a decrease in carotid artery blood flow of around 14 per cent (Tindall, Craddock and Greenfield, 1967). The effects of anaesthesia in the sitting position on organ systems other than the brain do not appear to have been documented.

Unless measures are taken to reduce the progressive pooling of blood into the lower part of the body there is transfer of fluid from the arteries and veins out into the extravascular tissues. This, therefore, reduces the blood volume still further. Measures to reduce these effects include bandaging the legs prior to positioning, the use of anti-gravity suits and external pneumatic compression apparatus applied to the lower limbs.

Air embolism

It is a well known clinical fact that when the surgical field is located significantly above the heart, air can be sucked in whenever a vein is partly or completely severed by the surgeon. Veins particularly at risk are those around and within the mastoid air cells because their walls are attached to the adjacent bone and they therefore remain open rather than collapsing. The major dural sinuses within the skull are similarly incapable of collapsing if inadvertently opened. The effects of posture on the pressure within the venous sinuses of the skull has been directly measured by Iwabuchi et al. (1983). They found that when the upper half of the body was raised, the confluens sinuum pressure decreased to reach zero at +25 degrees. When the angle was +90 degrees a marked negative pressure of $12.7 \pm 3.0\,cmH_2O$ (mean ± SD) was observed in adults. To obtain a confluens sinuum pressure of zero or a little higher the most favourable position is with the sinus 15 cm higher than the right atrium. In children under six years of age however such negative pressure was not observed even at an angle of +90 degrees.

Should a significant amount of air be allowed to enter the right ventricle of the heart the froth produced is unable to be cleared satisfactorily and cardiac arrest is a serious possibility.

Paradoxical air embolism

Under normal circumstances any small amounts of air entrained into the right side of the heart should not pass directly to the left heart but should be retained within the pulmonary circulation. Unfortunately, approximately 30 per cent of the population have a haemodynamically insignificant, but patent, foramen ovale, and when patients are anaesthetized in the sitting position the pressure in the left atrium can fall below that in the right (Perkins-Pearson, Marshall and Bedford, 1982). Under these circumstances, air can pass directly from the right to the left atrium and hence out into the systemic circulation. Although it has been proposed that lung ventilation with positive end-expiratory pressure (PEEP) could act both as a preventative measure to avoid air embolism and as acute treatment when embolism is suspected, Perkins and Bedford (1984) have shown that generally it impairs haemodynamic performance, it does not protect the patient against air embolism and it probably increases the risk of paradoxical air embolism in patients with probe-patent foramen ovale. Iwabuchi et al. (1983) also confirmed that PEEP does not raise the confluens sinuum pressure. Even very small bubbles of air can cause serious effects on entering the systemic side of the circulation, particularly if lodging in a branch of the cerebral circulation.

Change in posture as management of air embolism

On the basis of experiments in dogs it has long been recommended that patients should be changed rapidly from the sitting to the left lateral horizontal position to shift the obstructing bubble of air from the pulmonary outflow tract. However, a study of the anatomy in humans shows that it is the right lateral head-down position that places the pulmonary outflow tract inferior to the cavity of the ventricle. The early adoption of the left lateral position will, however, have the advantage of delaying the passage of air through the tricuspid valve into the right ventricle. It is likely that this manoeuvre would allow more time for the air that remains in the great veins and right atrium to be aspirated through an indwelling catheter (Leivers, Spilsbury and Young, 1971).

Summary of cardiorespiratory effects of the sitting position

The sitting position has little deleterious effect on the respiratory system irrespective of whether the patient has spontaneous respiration of intermittent positive pressure ventilation. In contrast, from the cardiovascular point of view, it presents the worst physiological trespass that any surgical patient must endure; with the added serious risk of air embolism.

Conclusion

Cardiovascular and respiratory changes resulting from anaesthesia and surgical posture probably can never be predicted accurately in any patient. It must always be assumed that there will be some adverse effects, and appropriate measures both to monitor and to correct them must be incorporated into the anaesthetic technique.

Anticipated malfunction of the respiratory system can usually be corrected by increasing the inspired oxygen levels and by substituting mechanical ventilation of the lungs for spontaneous breathing. Positive end-expiratory airway pressure can also be useful in some cases. Monitoring the results of these manoeuvres by the use of end-expired carbon dioxide measurement and intra-arterial gas sampling should present no difficulty. With the more widespread availability of transcutaneous oxygen saturation meters it will be even simpler.

The summated adverse effects of posture and anaesthesia on the cardiovascular system can be more difficult to manage. Careful preoperative assessment of the patient together with a considered and wise choice of anaesthetic drugs will pay dividends. Again, careful monitoring with a pulse meter, blood pressure recorder and electrocardiogram represent the minimum to be observed in any patient. There are some pharmacological agents which can be used to offset deleterious cardiovascular effects, but ultimately the posture itself might have to be modified in the best interests of the patient.

References

Altschule, M. D. and Zamcheck, N. (1942) Significance of changes in subdivisions of the lung volume in the Trendelenburg position. *Surgery, Gynecology and Obstetrics*, **74**, 1061–1064

Case, E. H. and Stiles, J. A. (1946) The effects of various surgical positions on vital capacity. *Anesthesiology*, **7**, 29–31

Chevrolet, J. C., Martin, J. G., Flood, R., Martin, R. R. and Engel, L. A. (1978) Topographical ventilation and perfusion distribution during IPPV in the lateral posture. *American Review of Respiratory Diseases*, **118**, 847–854

Coonan, T. J. and Hope, C. E. (1983) Cardiorespiratory effects of change of body position. *Canadian Anaesthetists Society Journal*, **30**, 424–437

Dalrymple, D. G., MacGowan, S. W. and MacLeod, G. F. (1979) Cardiorespiratory effects of the sitting position in neurosurgery. *British Journal of Anaesthesia*, **51**, 1079–1082

Denlinger, J. K., Kallos, T. and Marshall, B. E. (1972) Pulmonary blood flow distribution in man anesthetised in the lateral position. *Anesthesia and Analgesia Current Researches*, **51**, 260–263

Douglas, W. W., Rehder, K., Beynen, F. M., Sessler, A. D. and March, H. M. (1977) Improved oxygenation in patients with acute respiratory failure: the prone position. *American Review of Respiratory Diseases*, **115**, 559–566

Epstein, S. E., Stampfer, M. and Beiser, G. D. (1968) Role of the capacitance and resistance vessels in vasovagal syncope. *Circulation*, **37**, 524–533

Friberg, T. R. and Sandborn, G. (1985) Optic-nerve dysfunction during gravity inversion; pattern reversal evoked potentials. *Archives of Ophthalmology*, **103**, 1687–1689

Froese, A. B. and Bryan, A. C. (1974) Effects of anaesthesia and paralysis on diaphragmatic mechanics in man. *Anesthesiology*, **41**, 242–255

Guntheroth, W. G., Abel, F. L. and Mullins, G. L. (1964) The effect of Trendelenburg's position on blood pressure and carotid flow. *Surgery, Gynecology and Obstetrics*, **119**, 345–348

Iwabuchi, T., Sobata, E., Susuki, M., Susuki, S. and Yamashita, M. (1983) Dural sinus pressure as related to neurosurgical positions. *Neurosurgery*, **12**, 203–207

Leivers, D., Spilsbury, R. A. and Young, J. V. I. (1971) Air embolism during neurosurgery in the sitting position. Two case reports. *British Journal of Anaesthesia*, **43**, 84–89

Marshall, W. K., Bedford, R. F. and Miller, E. D. (1983) Cardiovascular responses in the seated position – impact of four anesthetic techniques. *Anesthesia and Analgesia*, **62**, 648–653

Perkins-Pearson, N. A. K., Marshall, W. K. and Bedford, R. F. (1982) Atrial pressures in the seated position. *Anesthesiology*, **57**, 493–497

Perkins, N. A. K. and Bedford, R. F. (1984) Hemodynamic consequences of PEEP in seated neurological patients – implications for paradoxical air embolism. *Anesthesia and Analgesia*, **63**, 429–432

Piehl, M. A. and Brown, R. S. (1976) Use of extreme position changes in acute respiratory failure. *Critical Care Medicine*, **4**, 13–14

Reed, J. H. Jr. and Wood, E. H. (1970) Effect of body position on vertical distribution of pulmonary blood flow. *Journal of Applied Physiology*, **28**, 303–311

Rehder, K., Hatch, D. J., Sessler, A. D. and Ward, S. F. (1972) The function of each lung of anesthetised and paralysed man during mechanical ventilation. *Anesthesiology*, **37(i)**, 16–26

Rehder, K. and Sessler, A. D. (1973) Function of each lung in spontaneously breathing man anaesthetised with thiopental–meperidine. *Anesthesiology*, **38**, 320–327

Scott, D. B., Lees, M. M. and Taylor, S. H. (1966) Some respiratory effects of the Trendelenburg position during anaesthesia. *British Journal of Anaesthesia*, **38**, 174–178

Shenkin, H. A., Scheuerman, E. B., Spitz, E. B. and Groff, R. A. (1949) Effect of change of posture upon cerebral circulation of man. *Journal of Applied Physiology*, **2**, 317–326

Sibbald, W. J., Patterson, N. A. M., Holliday, R. L. and Baskeville, J. (1979) The Trendelenburg position: Hemodynamic effects in hypotensive and normotensive patients. *Critical Care Medicine*, **7**, 218–224

Snoy, F. J. and Woodside, J. R. (1984) Unilateral pulmonary oedema (down lung syndrome) following urological operation. *Journal of Urology*, **132**, 776–777

Stone, J. E. and Khambatta, H. J. (1978) Pulmonary shunts in the prone position. *Anaesthesia*, **33**, 512–517

Tarkkanen, A. and Leikola, J. (1967) Postural variations of the intra-ocular pressure as measured with the Mackay–Marg Tonometer. *Acta Ophthalmologica*, **45**, 569–575

Taylor, J. and Weil, M. H. (1967) Failure of the Trendelenburg position to improve circulation during clinical shock. *Surgery, Gynecology and Obstetrics*, **124**, 1005–1010

Tindall, G. T., Craddock, A. and Greenfield, J. C. (1967) Effects of the sitting position on blood flow in the internal carotid artery of man during general anaesthesia. *Journal of Neurosurgery*, **26**, 383–389

Weil, M. H., MacLean, L. D., Visscher, M. B. and Spink, W. W. (1956) Studies on the circulatory changes in the dog produced by endotoxin from gram negative organisms. *Journal of Clinical Investigation*, **35**, 1191–1197

Weil, M. H. and Whigham, H. (1965) Head-down (Trendelenburg) position for treatment of irreversible haemorrhagic shock. Experimental study in rats. *Annals of Surgery*, **162**, 905–909

West, J. B. (1974) *Respiratory Physiology – the Essentials*, pp. 41–43. Williams & Wilkins Company, Baltimore

Wilkins, R. W., Bradley, S. E. and Friedland, C. K. (1950) The acute circulatory effects of the head down position (negative G) in normal man with a note on some measures to relieve cranial congestion in this position. *Journal of Clinical Investigation*, **29**, 940–949

Index

Page numbers in *italic* type indicate illustration(s), or text and illustration(s) occurring on the same page